The 101 Healthiest Foods for Kids

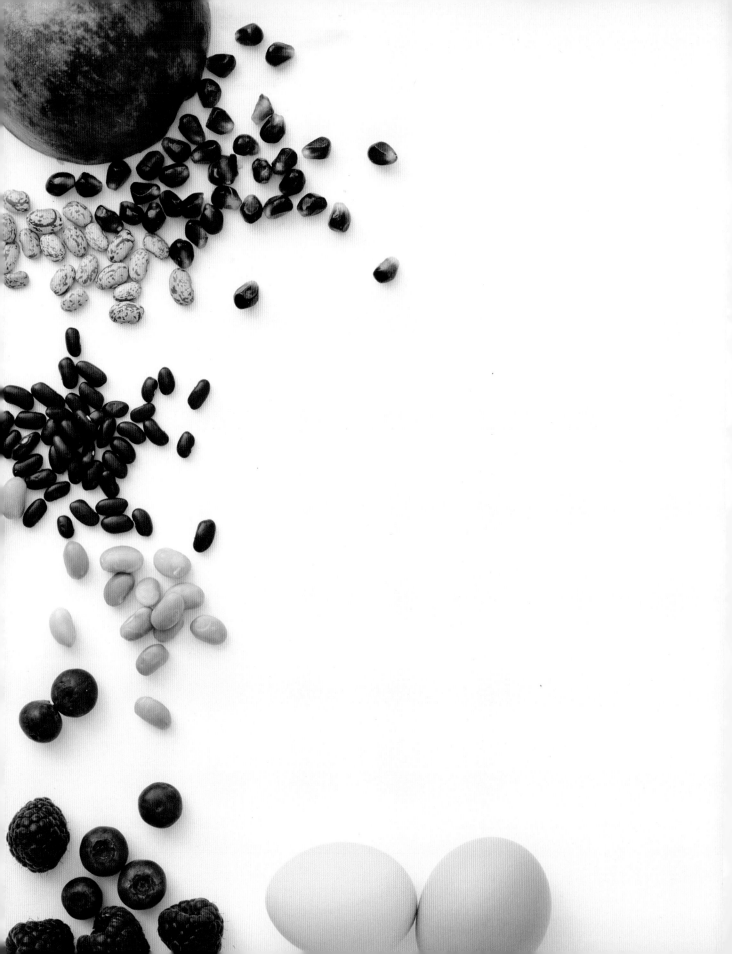

The 101 Healthiest Foods for Kids

Eat the Best, Feel the Greatest—
Healthy Foods for Kids, and Recipes Too

Sally Kuzemchak, M.S., R.D.

FAIR WINDS

Brimming with creative inspiration, how-to projects, and useful information to enrich your everyday life, Quarto Knows is a favorite destination for those pursuing their interests and passions. Visit our site and dig deeper with our books into your area of interest: Quarto Creates, Quarto Cooks, Quarto Homes, Quarto Lives, Quarto Drives, Quarto Explores, Quarto Gifts, or Quarto Kids.

First Published in 2019 by Fair Winds Press, an imprint of The Quarto Group,
100 Cummings Center, Suite 265-D, Beverly, MA 01915, USA.
T (978) 282-9590 F (978) 283-2742 QuartoKnows.com

Fair Winds Press titles are also available at discount for retail, wholesale, promotional, and bulk purchase. For details, contact the Special Sales Manager by email at specialsales@quarto.com or by mail at The Quarto Group, Attn: Special Sales Manager, 401 Second Avenue North, Suite 310, Minneapolis, MN 55401, USA.

23 22 21 20 19   1 2 3 4 5

ISBN: 978-1-59233-848-1

Digital edition published in 2019
eISBN: 978-1-63159-538-7

Library of Congress Cataloging-in-Publication Data available.

Design: Rita Sowins / Sowins Design
Cover Image: Glenn Scott Photography
Page Layout: Rita Sowins / Sowins Design
Photography: Glenn Scott Photography and Shutterstock

Printed in China

The information in this book is for educational purposes only. It is not intended to replace the advice of a physician or medical practitioner.

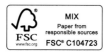

For my guys:
Joel,
Henry, and
Sam

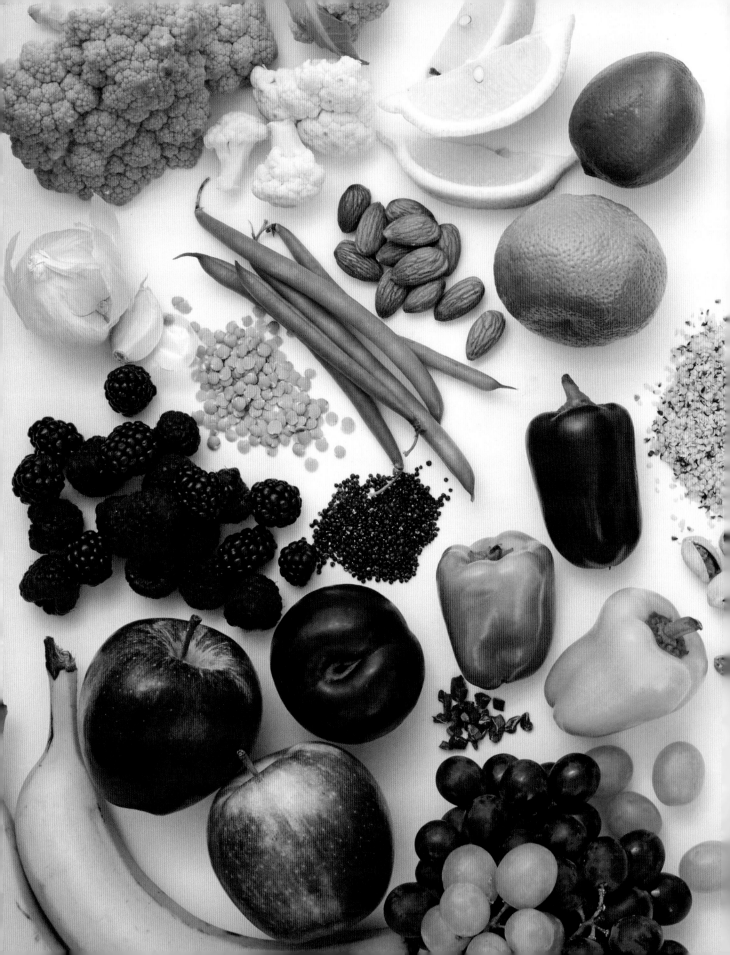

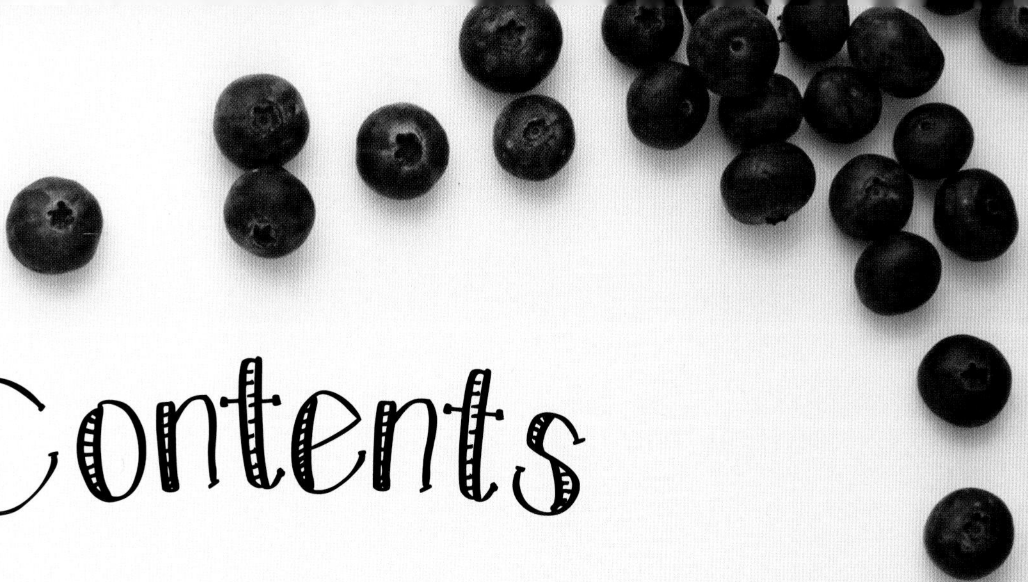

Contents

Introduction 12

1: Vegetables 17

2: Fruits 67

3: Grains 115

4: Protein-Rich Foods 135

5: Spices & Seasonings 177

Top 10 Lists 192
Resources 200
Acknowledgments 201
About the Author 202
Index 203

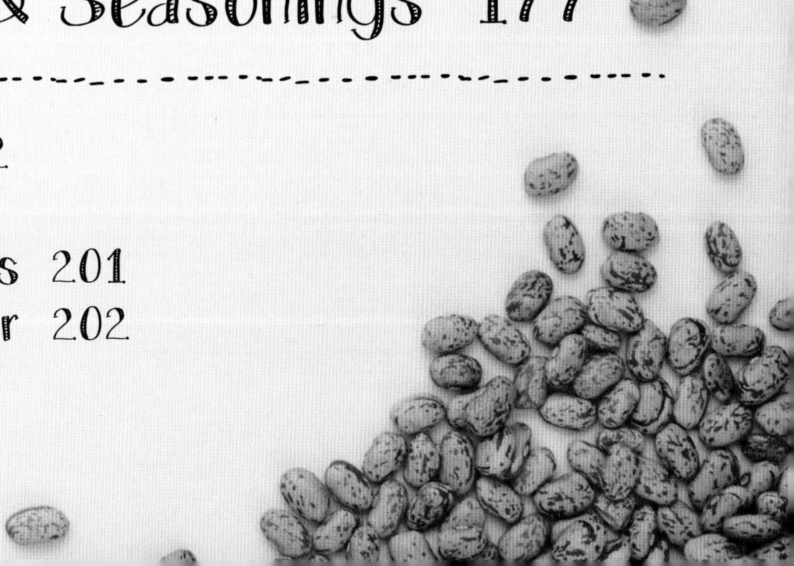

The 101 Healthiest Foods, By Chapter

Chapter 1: Vegetables

1: Asparagus . . . 18

2: Beets (Recipe: Berry and Beet Smoothie) . . . 20

3: Broccoli (Recipe: Game-Changing Roasted Broccoli) . . . 22

4: Brussels Sprouts (Recipe: Cheesy Brussels Sprouts Chips) . . . 24

5: Butternut Squash . . . 26

6+7: Cabbage + Sauerkraut . . . 28

8: Carrots (Recipe: Sweet Carrot Salad) . . . 30

9: Cauliflower (Recipe: Cauliflower Nuggets) . . . 32

10: Celery . . . 34

11: Corn (Recipe: Brown Bag Popcorn) . . . 36

12: Cucumbers . . . 38

13: Eggplant . . . 40

14: Green Beans . . . 42

15: Green Peas . . . 44

16: Jicama . . . 45

17: Kale (Recipe: Crunchy Kale Chips) . . . 46

18: Kohlrabi . . . 48

19: Mushrooms . . . 49

20: Onions . . . 50

21: Potatoes . . . 52

22: Pumpkin (Recipe: Pumpkin Chocolate Chip Pancakes) . . . 54

23: Romaine Lettuce . . . 56

24: Spinach . . . 57

25: Sweet Peppers . . . 58

26: Sweet Potatoes . . . 60

27: Tomatoes . . . 62

28: Zucchini . . . 64

Chapter 2: Fruits

29: Apples . . . 68

30: Apricots . . . 70

31: Avocados (Recipe: Starter Guacamole) . . . 72

32: Bananas (Recipe: Blueberry Banana "Ice Cream") . . . 74

33+34: Blackberries + Raspberries . . . 76

35+36: Blueberries + Wild Blueberries . . . 78

37+38: Cantaloupe + Honeydew . . . 80

39: Cherries . . . 82

40: Coconut . . . 84

41: Dates . . . 86

42: Grapefruit (Recipe: Broiled Grapefruit) . . . 88

43+44: Grapes + Raisins . . . 90

45: Kiwi . . . 92

46+47: Lemons + Limes . . . 93

48: Papaya . . . 94

49: Mango . . . 95

50: Olives . . . 96

51: Oranges (Recipe: Better-for-You Orange Julius) . . . 98

52: Peaches . . . 100

53: Pears . . . 102

54: Pineapple . . . 104

55+56: Plums + Prunes . . . 106

57: Pomegranate . . . 108

58: Strawberries (Recipe: Melted Berry Sauce) . . . 110

59: Watermelon . . . 112

Chapter 3: Grains

60: Barley . . . 116

61: Brown Rice . . . 118

62: Bulgur . . . 120

63: Couscous . . . 122

64: Farro . . . 124

65: Millet . . . 125

66: Oats (Recipe: Make-Ahead Instant Oatmeal Packets) . . . 126

67: Quinoa (Recipe: Baked Quinoa Bites) . . . 128

68: Whole Wheat (Recipe: Homemade Tortillas) . . . 130

69: Wild Rice . . . 132

Chapter 4: Protein-Rich Foods

70: Beans . . . 136

71: Beef . . . 137

72: Chickpeas (Recipe: Taco-Spiced Skillet Chickpeas) . . . 138

73: Cottage Cheese . . . 140

74: Kefir . . . 142

75: Milk . . . 144

76: Yogurt (Recipe: Very Berry Pops) . . . 146

77: Edamame . . . 148

78: Eggs . . . 150

79: Lentils (Recipe: Red Lentil Snack Cookies) . . . 152

80: Pistachios . . . 155

81: Almonds . . . 156

82: Peanuts (Recipe: Homemade Peanut Butter) . . . 158

83: Walnuts . . . 160

84: Chia Seeds . . . 162

85: Flaxseed . . . 163

86: Hemp Seeds . . . 164

87: Sunflower Seeds (Recipe: Nut-Free Snack Balls) . . . 166

88: Tahini (Recipe: Easy Peasy Hummus) . . . 168

89: Salmon . . . 170

90: Tofu (Recipe: Speedy Miso Noodle Soup) . . . 172

91: Tuna . . . 174

Chapter 5: Spices & Seasonings

92+93: Chocolate + Cocoa (Recipe: Chocolate Breakfast Shake) . . . 178

94: Cinnamon . . . 180

95: Garlic (Recipe: Easy Peanut Sauce) . . . 182

96: Ginger . . . 184

97: Honey . . . 185

98: Nutritional Yeast . . . 186

99: Olive Oil . . . 187

100: Oregano (Recipe: Homemade Pizza Sauce) . . . 188

101: Turmeric . . . 190

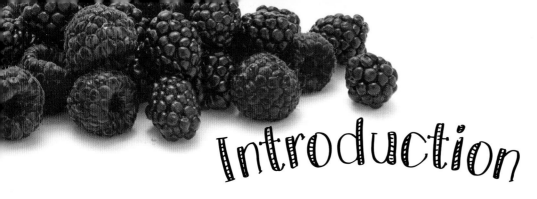

Introduction

"What should I feed my kid?"

I get that question a lot.

As a dietitian who focuses on family nutrition, I hear from parents every day who are determined to feed their kids the healthiest diet possible. But they're up against the challenges of balancing life with kids, including finicky eaters and busy schedules—not to mention maddeningly conflicting information about what healthy eating even means. Between what you hear from your Facebook feed, moms on the playground, and the random person behind you in line at the grocery store, it's enough to confuse anyone.

The reality is that there's no single prescription for growing a healthy child. But there's definitely a pattern of eating that's strongly linked in research to healthier, longer lives. This includes plenty of fruits and vegetables, whole grains, lean proteins, and healthy fats. Those foods are exactly what this book is all about.

Why You Need This Book

Raise your hand if you obsessed over those very first spoonfuls when your child started solids. (I sure did!) Most parents bend over backward to make sure their babies have a balance of green and orange vegetables, a mix of fruits, and nourishing finger foods. No wonder government surveys find that most babies have top-notch nutrition, with intakes of vitamins and minerals that meet or exceed what they need.

Then something happens.

Babies grow into toddlers and then preschoolers, and picky eating sets in. They discover gummy fruit snacks and cookies. Eating habits take a nosedive. The most popular vegetable becomes potatoes—in the form of french fries. Whole grains plummet, and sweets are on the rise. On a given day, a third of preschoolers don't get a single serving of vegetables and a quarter of pre-schoolers don't eat a bite of fruit. And things don't improve as they get older and gain more independence and influence over their food choices. During adolescence, a time when kids need calcium the most, soda and other sugary drinks start to replace milk.

In other words, kids' habits need help. Not just because children require a nutrient-rich diet to grow and thrive, but also because habits developed during childhood can have a lasting impact on eating into adulthood.

The good news: Whether you've got a toddler or a teen, it's never too late to turn habits around.

What's So Great about These Foods

I'd never tell you to make everything from scratch or avoid anything in a package. I know that some convenience foods are a reality for most families, including my own. But whole foods should form the foundation of your child's day. This book offers 101 places to start.

Sure, there are plenty of healthy foods that didn't make the cut—and by all means, keep serving them! But there's no denying that certain foods stand out, not only because they're rich in nutrients that many kids are missing out on—like fiber, potassium, magnesium, and vitamin D—but also because they're abundant in natural compounds proven to help safeguard your child's health.

The Best Way to Use This Book

Sit down and flip through this book with your kids. You'll spot some foods that are already regulars on your plates, and I'll give you even more reasons to keep them there—plus some new ways to serve them. You'll also see foods you've attempted to serve in the past and abandoned, and I'll make the case for trying again (and again). And you may even find foods that are totally unfamiliar. I'll walk you through why you should give them a shot, plus how to select, prep, and serve them. And throughout, I've sprinkled fun facts about the foods that make for great dinner conversation.

HOW TO ENCOURAGE KIDS TO TRY NEW FOODS

Do:

• Model healthy eating habits. Let your kids see you eating and enjoying healthy foods.

• Make it fun. Have your kids create a star chart to record all the new foods they've tried or enlist them as new food "reviewers" and ask for ratings on taste, texture, and smell.

• Try new approaches. Serve foods cooked in different ways, cut into different shapes, and flavored with different seasonings.

• Allow your child to (politely) spit out a food they have tasted but don't like.

Don't:

- Force your children to eat foods they don't want to eat.

- Bribe your child with a promise of dessert if she tries a new food.

- Sneak or hide foods like vegetables in their meals. Be truthful about what's in the dish. (Better yet, have them help you make it!)

- Call your child "picky." Labeling your child in this way isn't helpful and won't encourage her to be brave and adventurous.

And in Case You're Wondering . . .

Don't worry: My feet are firmly planted in reality. I know that magic doesn't always happen when you serve new foods. And despite endless articles telling you that kids will try a food after 10 to 15 exposures, I know some kids still won't budge after 25 tries. That's why I made sure to include "Try It" tips along the way with gentle, nonthreatening ways to present unfamiliar foods to reluctant eaters. You'll also get answers to some of your biggest questions when it comes to feeding kids—plus some reassuring words if you're currently freaking out over a kid who won't drink a drop of milk or touch a single veggie.

If you want to know whether *my* kids eat every one of these 101 foods, *yeah right*! I may be a dietitian, but I've still got pretty typical kids who can be stubborn about stepping outside their comfort zones (and who never met a bowl of mac and cheese they didn't like). But no matter what, I always maintain hope. After all, my thirteen-year-old swore he didn't like chickpeas until he tried the Taco-Spiced Skillet Chickpeas (page 139). And my nine-year-old fell in love with pomegranate seeds after seeing friends at school gobble them up at lunchtime.

The moral of the story: Never stop trying. Your kids (and their health) are worth it.

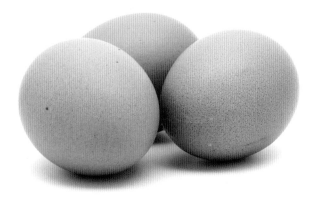
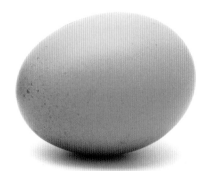

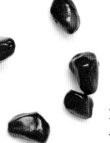

MY TEN HEALTHY EATING RULES TO LIVE (AND FEED) BY

1. Serve regular meals and snacks. When kids can depend on meals and snacks served regularly throughout the day, they're less likely to mindlessly graze or overeat.

2. Offer a fruit and/or vegetable at most meals and snacks. Kids (and grown-ups) don't get nearly enough fruits and vegetables. If you make an effort to serve them at most meals and snacks, your family is more likely to get what they need.

3. Pour water and milk most often. Sweet drinks are the number one source of added sugar for kids and adults. Save them for special occasions or once in a while when you're out to eat.

4. Stock the kitchen with healthy foods. The outside world is full of soda, chips, and candy. Occasional treats are okay, but make healthy foods the default in your home.

5. Prepare just one meal. Don't be a short-order cook. Plan one dinner each night for the whole family, but be sure there are at least one or two items on the table that you know your child likes (even if it's just a favorite veggie or dinner rolls).

6. Involve your child. Kids who take part in food prep are more likely to feel invested and proud of the meal—so they're more likely to eat it and enjoy it. If they're not helping in the kitchen, offer them choices when you can that give them ownership: Roasted broccoli or cooked carrots? Brown rice or couscous?

7. Be neutral about dessert. Avoid bribing kids with the promise of dessert or withholding it as a punishment for not eating enough.

8. Eat together as often as possible. Research shows that kids who eat with their families more often take in more nutrients and are better off socially and emotionally. Family dinner may not work every night, but gather together as much as possible.

9. Focus on a happy table. Keep mealtime a positive environment so your child feels relaxed and accepted at the table.

10. Let it go. Don't count how many bites your child takes of her broccoli or stress out if she eats only bread for one meal. It's your child's overall eating that counts, not one individual meal, day, or even week that matters.

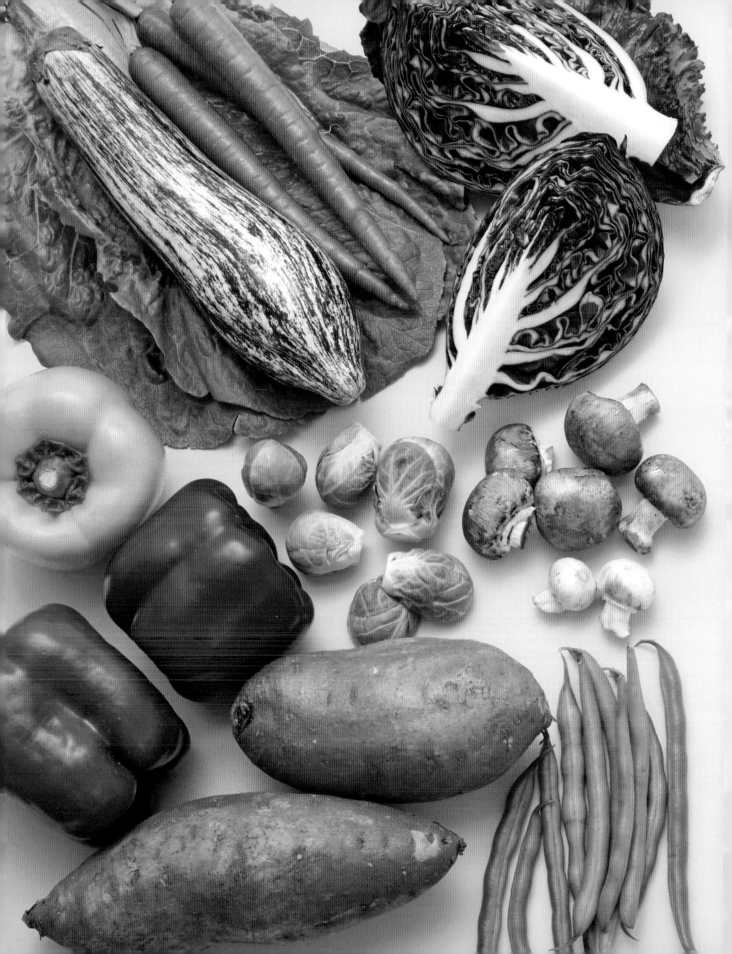

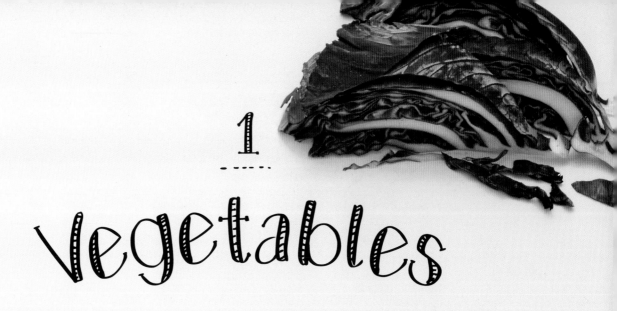

1

Vegetables

Vegetables have a lot going for them. They're rich in vitamins A and C, fiber, and plant compounds that help guard against disease. They're also hydrating and low in calories. Developing a love of veggies and a habit of eating them regularly will serve your kids well throughout their entire lives. If only it were that easy.

Truth is, vegetables are a source of angst for many parents and kids. Unlike fruit, most veggies aren't very sweet, and some can be downright bitter (I'm looking at you, kale). And too often, veggies are overcooked, rendering them mushy, unappetizing, and ideal for secretly feeding to the dog under the table. After one too many wrinkled noses at the dinner table, many parents simply throw in the towel. It's no wonder that children of every age group are falling short on their daily needs—and that the most beloved and commonly eaten vegetable among kids is the french fry.

The mission: to transform your kids' attitudes about vegetables from "Yuck!" to "Yum!" or at least "Sure, I'll have a bite" (we'll also take "I'm not going to eat it, but I don't mind it being on my plate" because for some kids, that's progress too!). The key to doing this is to offer vegetables every day—lots of different kinds in lots of different ways. Sure, not every single one will be a smashing success, but stay the course and you may just stumble on some new favorites.

HOW MANY VEGETABLES DO YOUR KIDS NEED EVERY DAY?

- Ages 2–3: 1 cup*
- Ages 4–8: 1½ cups*
- Ages 9–13: 2 cups (girls), 2½ cups (boys)*
- Ages 14–18: 2½ cups (girls), 3 cups (boys)*

*Weight varies. Source: United States Department of Agriculture (USDA)

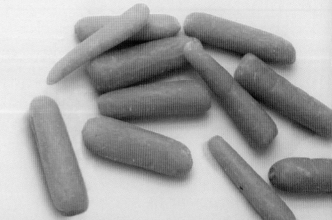

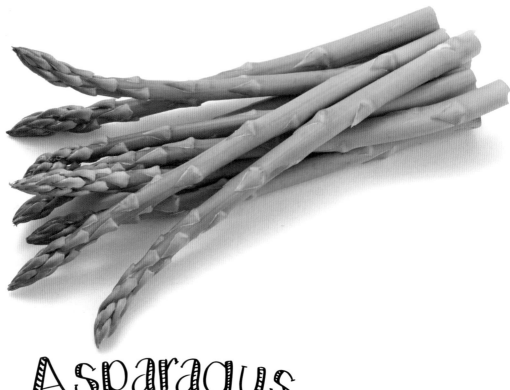

Asparagus

This veggie can do a lot for kids nutritionally. One cup (125 g) of chopped spears has a third of the **folate, vitamin C,** and **iron** that young children need in a day. It also packs in their **whole day's worth of vitamin K,** which helps blood clot after a cut and helps the body absorb calcium so it can build bone. Asparagus is also a **powerhouse source of antioxidants** such as rutin, a compound that's being studied for positive effects on memory and body weight.

But let's be real: Your kid will probably be a lot more interested in the Stinky Pee Effect. That's what happens to some people after eating asparagus, when the veggie's asparagusic acid converts to sulfur-containing compounds, giving the urine a distinctive (and not very pleasant) odor. It can take effect as quickly as 15 minutes after the asparagus is eaten—but it doesn't seem to happen to everyone. Whether that's because not everyone produces stinky asparagus pee or only certain people can detect the smell is unknown. But whatever the reason, it definitely makes for a somewhat silly after-dinner experiment!

Asparagus is a spring veggie and can be pricey outside the growing season, so get the fresh stuff while you can. When choosing asparagus, look for tips that are dark green or purple and very tightly packed and closed (the tips start to wilt and open when it gets old). Once it's home, store the bunch in the refrigerator, upright in a glass with some water covering the bottoms.

The key to cooking asparagus right is to not overcook it. Over-cooked spears will get limp and wimpy, so cook it quickly (such as in a speedy sauté or roast) to preserve its firm texture and bright green hue. Even though cooking decreases the vitamin C content some, it boosts the activity of antioxidants, natural compounds that offer disease protection.

HOW TO TRIM ASPARAGUS

The ends of asparagus spears are tough and woody. To remove that part, gently bend each spear until it snaps. Or you can trim the spears at the point where the color changes from white to green.

Good to Know

Rumors have been circulating online for years that puréed asparagus can cure cancer, thanks to its rich supply of glutathione, a substance that protects cells from damage. That claim has been debunked, but take heart: Nutrients found in asparagus, such as folate, vitamin C, and beta-carotene, still offer some cancer protection, according to the American Institute for Cancer Research.

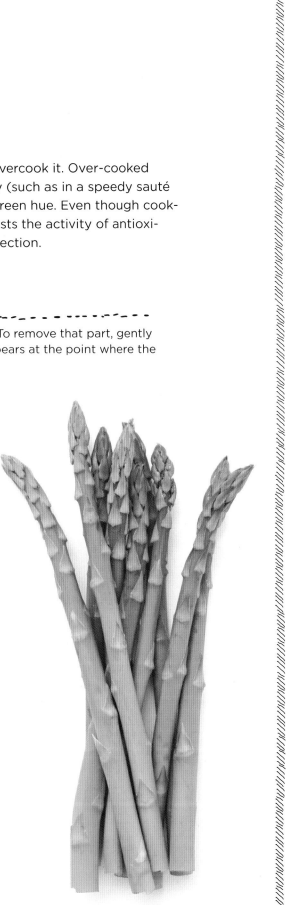

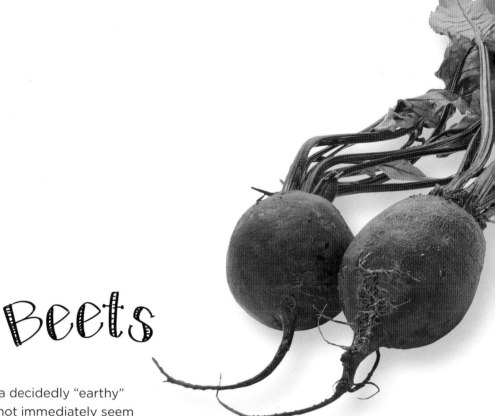

Beets

Yes, beets have a decidedly "earthy" flavor that may not immediately seem kid-friendly. But beets are also rich in natural sugars, making them sweeter than many other veggies. Golden beets have the most sugar, so they're a good bet for first-time beet-eaters. You may also want to casually mention to your kids that their pee and poop may turn red after they eat beets. For a certain kind of kid (and you know if you've got one!), that just might do the trick.

Beets are a root veggie, and they're entirely edible—from the root to the greens on top. You'll find beets in shades of red and gold, as well as some with pink and white stripes. A half cup of beets is a **great source of potassium, folate, vitamin B$_6$, and vitamin C** for kids and has a couple grams of fiber. The leafy tops are rich in beta-carotene and contain both calcium and iron. The pigments that color red and pink beets are called betalains and are used by the food industry as a natural food coloring. In the body, betalains work as antioxidants and are also being studied for their ability to **inhibit cancer cells and microbes such as *E. coli* and salmonella** and **lower cholesterol**.

Once you get beets home from the store, trim off the greens, leaving an inch (2.5 cm) of the stem intact, and place them unwashed in a plastic bag for up to three weeks (store the greens in a bag as well and use within a few days). You can thinly slice beets and roast them to make baked beet "chips." If your kids like pickles, try pickled beets. They taste similar to pickles, so they may seem more familiar. Use the tops the same way you'd use spinach in recipes.

Berry and Beet Smoothie

My older son, who isn't game for eating cooked beets yet, happily slurps down a certain berry and beet smoothie served at a local neighborhood lunch spot. He gives the thumbs-up to this copy-cat version too.

½ cup (75 g) fresh or frozen strawberries
½ cup (80 g) frozen blueberries
1 small banana (or ½ large banana)
½ small beet, chopped
½ cup (120 ml) almond milk (or dairy milk)
2 teaspoons honey

Place the strawberries, blueberries, banana, beet, milk, and honey in a high-speed blender in the order listed. Blend until smooth and serve immediately.

Yield: 2 servings

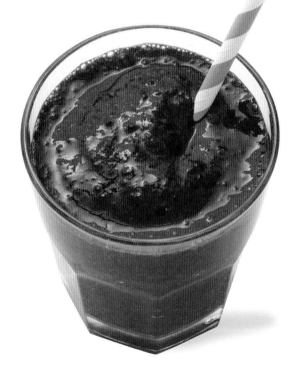

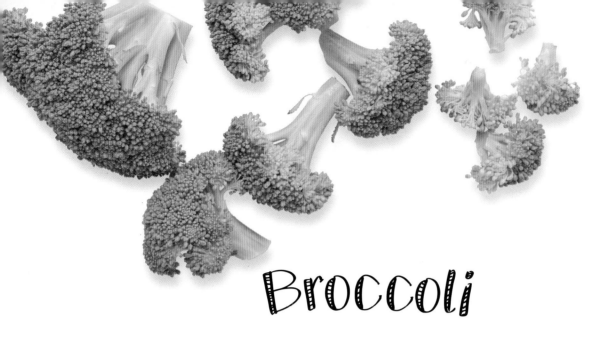

Broccoli

If you're a parent, you've probably uttered the words "eat your broccoli." Though I'm not a fan of nagging kids to eat anything, I get it. And truth be told, broccoli is worthy of the effort. A cruciferous vegetable, broccoli is part of the Brassica family (along with its cousins cabbage, cauliflower, and Brussels sprouts) and contains plant chemicals that are known to be **natural cancer fighters**. A half-cup (35 g) serving of broccoli has **as much vitamin C as half of an orange**, plus folate, vitamin A, and even **a little bit of protein and calcium**.

Broccoli comes from a Latin word meaning "branch," and calling the florets "trees" just might be enough to get a smile (and a nibble) from reluctant kids. When buying broccoli, choose deep-colored florets in dark green or even purple. They're richer in vitamins than lighter ones. Avoid yellowed broccoli, which is a sign of age. And remember that you don't have to throw away the broccoli stalks. Just peel away the tough outer part, cut them into sticks, salt them, and serve them raw. Or toss raw chunks into green salads, bake them into casseroles along with the florets, or use them to flavor homemade broth.

Though some kids like raw broccoli, it can be slightly bitter that way. Cooking it quickly just until it's "tender-crisp" (so it is soft but has some bite) and still bright green will make the flavor less sharp and may even provide some additional health benefits. One study published in the *Journal of Agricultural and Food Chemistry* found that steaming broccoli actually increased the antioxidant concentration by as much as 30 percent compared to raw. Be careful not to overcook it, though; this can discolor the broccoli and increase nutrient loss. The slight odor you get when cooking broccoli is from sulfurous chemicals called glucosinolates, which form compounds in the body that may inhibit the growth of some kinds of cancers, according to the National Cancer Institute.

Game-Changing Roasted Broccoli

Obviously, broccoli won't wow any kid if it's overcooked and mushy. This is why roasting broccoli is a game-changer for many parents when it comes to convincing picky eaters. Roasting brings out broccoli's natural sweetness.

4 cups (280 g) raw broccoli florets
1 tablespoon (15 ml) olive oil
½ teaspoon garlic salt
¼ cup (25 g) grated or shredded Parmesan cheese

Preheat the oven to 425°F (220°C) and line a baking sheet with parchment paper. In a medium bowl, toss the broccoli with the oil. Sprinkle with the garlic salt and toss again. Scatter the broccoli in a single layer on the baking sheet and roast for 15 minutes, or until it reaches the desired brownness. Return the broccoli to the same bowl, sprinkle with the Parmesan cheese, and toss well. Serve immediately.

Yield: 4 servings

"TRY IT" TIP

Let them dunk! In a study published in the *Journal of the Academy of Nutrition and Dietetics*, preschoolers who were especially sensitive to bitter flavors ate 80 percent more broccoli at snack time when it was served alongside ranch dressing than they did when it was served plain.

BROCCOLINI

It's sometimes called baby broccoli, but it's actually a hybrid—a cross between regular broccoli and Chinese broccoli. It's packed with vitamins A and C and a bit of iron. With longer, skinnier stalks, broccolini tastes similar to regular broccoli (sometimes a bit sweeter) and can be prepped and served the same way.

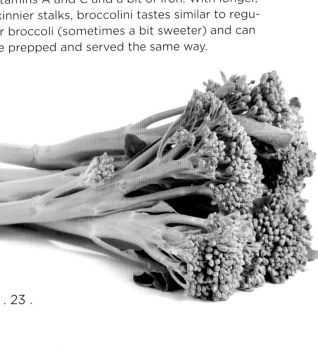

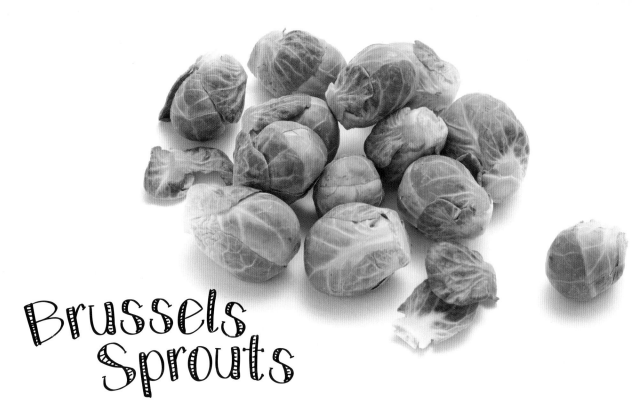

Brussels Sprouts

Has any other vegetable earned a worse reputation than Brussels sprouts? In books and popular media, they're practically shorthand for "yucky food kids don't want to eat." You may even have your own childhood scars from facing down a sad pile of sprouts and not being allowed to leave the table until you took a bite. But gone are the days of boiling Brussels into a bitter mush. We now know that they really shine when they're roasted to bring out their sweetness or sautéed with chunks of apples (or, hello, bacon!).

Brussels sprouts are finally having a moment, and these little cabbages deserve their time in the spotlight. A half-cup (44 g) serving packs a **whole day's worth of vitamin C** for young kids, plus some **fiber and protein**. As with other cruciferous vegetables such as broccoli and cauliflower, Brussels sprouts may offer some cancer protection thanks to sulfur-containing chemicals (which explains the odor when cooking!) that are broken down during digestion into beneficial compounds. These compounds have been shown in animal studies to prevent the growth of cancers like breast, colon, and lung. Though this hasn't been proven in human research, there's no doubt that cruciferous veggies should have a spot on your child's plate.

If you have a farmers' market nearby, stop by in the fall or early winter when Brussels sprouts are in season and see if you can snag a whole stalk. Your kids will get a kick out of how the little cabbages grow in a tight, circular pattern around a long, thick stem.

➡ Cheesy Brussels Sprouts Chips

No matter how trendy, Brussels sprouts are still a hard sell for some kids (and grown-ups!), so consider this a "bridge" recipe. Serving these crispy chips can help a picky eater become familiar with Brussels sprouts—and maybe even nudge them along to whole sprouts eventually. This is also a handy way to use all the leaves that fall off the sprouts when you're slicing them.

12 ounces (340 g) Brussels sprouts
1 teaspoon olive oil
Pinch of salt
¼ teaspoon nutritional yeast

Preheat the oven to 275°F (140°C) and line a baking sheet with parchment paper or aluminum foil. Remove stems from the Brussels sprouts, then peel off the outer leaves (this is a great job for kids!) until you have about 2 cups (110 g) of loosely packed leaves. Toss the leaves with olive oil and salt and place in a single layer on the baking sheet. Bake for 10 to 12 minutes, or until crisp. Sprinkle with the nutritional yeast and serve immediately.

Yield: 2 servings

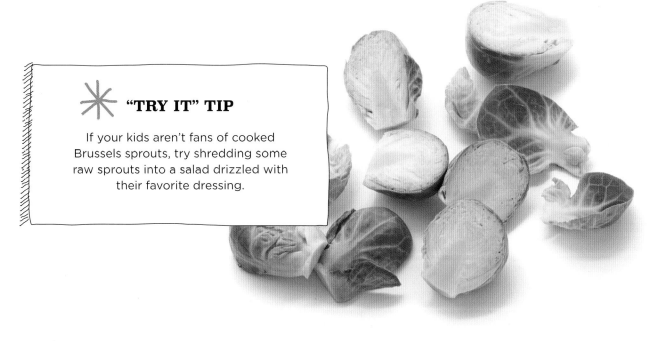

✳ "TRY IT" TIP

If your kids aren't fans of cooked Brussels sprouts, try shredding some raw sprouts into a salad drizzled with their favorite dressing.

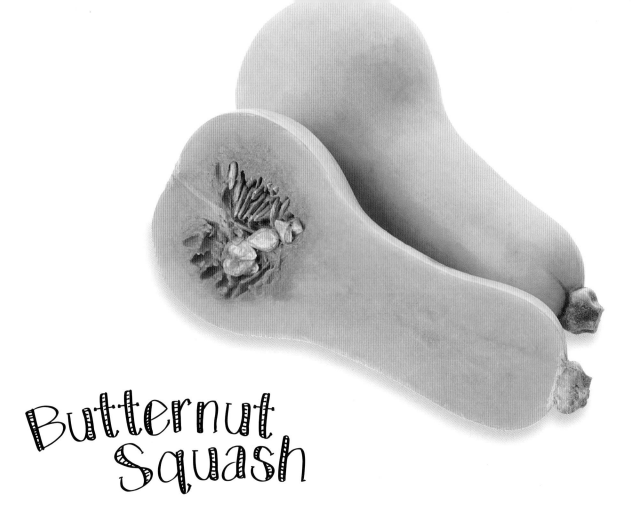

Butternut Squash

Squash is one of those veggies that's a mainstay on high chair trays but can fall by the wayside as kids get older (and more finicky). But it's worth circling back to squash such as butternut, acorn, and summer because they're all healthy in their own ways. Butternut has the distinction of tasting slightly sweet, which may be more appealing to kids. The dark orange flesh means it's **loaded with beta-carotene**, a pigment that works as an antioxidant in the body. The squash also contains another carotenoid called beta-cryptoxanthin, which is linked to both a lower risk for lung cancer and inflammatory arthritis. It's also **packed with vitamin A and folate** (a B vitamin that helps build new cells) plus some potassium, vitamin C, and a **couple grams of fiber** to boot.

When squash shopping, choose one that is heavy for its size and has no blemishes or green patches on its skin. Buy the size you need; a large squash doesn't mean it's less flavorful or nutritious than a small one. Once home, squash keeps well for weeks in a cool, dry place. When you're ready to use it, remove the skin with a vegetable peeler (that's easier to do if you first cut apart the wide "bulb" end from the "neck" end). Slice the bulb in half and scoop out the seeds with a spoon. Then you can cube it and roast it along with sweet potatoes and other veggies.

You can also bake the whole squash for purée. Here's how: Leaving the skin on, cut the squash in half and scoop out the seeds with a spoon. Rub some olive oil on the flesh and roast it, cut-side down, on a baking sheet at 400°F (200°C) until it's really soft and can be pierced easily with a fork (check it after thirty minutes, though it may take up to an hour for a very large squash). You can scoop out the purée (with a spoon or ice cream scoop) to use in soups, quick bread, or any recipe that calls for pumpkin purée. Your kids may also enjoy a bowl of sweet butternut squash soup that's made with puréed apple.

Good to Know

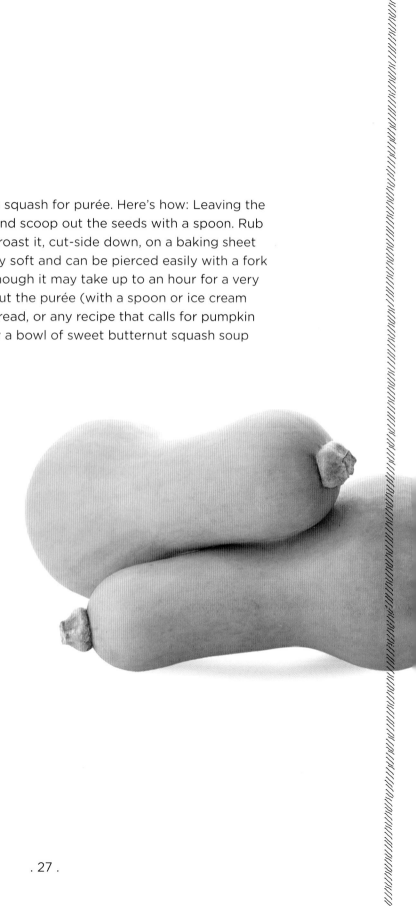

Veggies taste better when they're fresh, so follow these tips:

- On your refrigerator's crisper drawer, choose "high humidity" for leafy greens.

- Store veggies such as asparagus and green onions upright in a jar of water (like you would flowers in a vase).

- Keep potatoes, onions, and squash on the counter or in the pantry.

- Got limp carrots and celery? Wash and slice them and place in a container of cold water. They'll absorb some of the water and become crisp again.

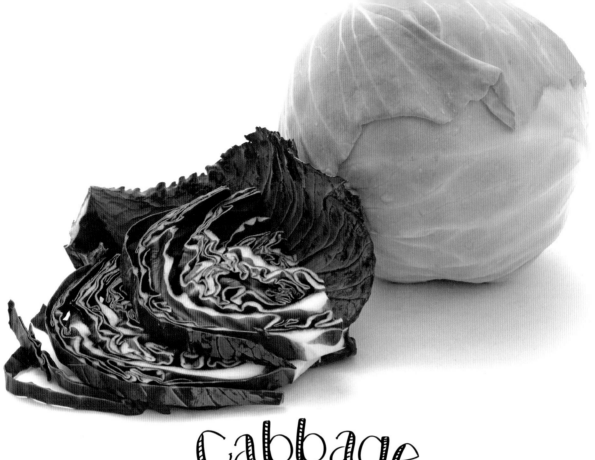

Cabbage

Don't be fooled into thinking that cabbage is a nutritional lightweight like iceberg lettuce. As a member of the famed Brassica family along with broccoli and kale, this humble, budget-friendly veggie boasts **potent cancer-fighting compounds**. Cabbage is **rich in vitamin C and is a good source of fiber**, and it has a little bit of calcium and potassium too. Red cabbage has bonus disease-fighting powers thanks to anthocyanins, the plant pigments that create its purple-red hue (they're the same ones found in blueberries), and a bit more vitamin C.

Some kids like cabbage leaves stuffed with flavorful ground meat, rice, and veggies. If your child is iffy on cooked cabbage (the smell *can* be a little strong), try stirring small shreds of Napa cabbage into colorful stir-fries toward the end of cooking. Raw cabbage is also great for kids because of its crunch, so try adding thinly sliced red or purple cabbage to green salads (add just a few slices at a time to start). My kids also like raw purple cabbage tucked into fish tacos on little flour tortillas. Or make a bright slaw from red and green cabbage, thinly sliced apples, and dressing. Try to slice cabbage just before serving to reduce the amount of vitamin loss.

Q: Is it Okay to Make My Child a Separate Meal if She Doesn't Like What We're Having?

It's understandable that so many parents end up doing this—after all, you want your child to eat *something* for dinner! But this is a habit you should break. Being a short-order cook isn't good for you (who has time to cook multiple dinners?) or your kids, who will never learn to try new foods if they're served old familiars every night. Aim to serve just one meal each night, making sure you have at least one or two foods on the table that you know your child will reliably eat, even if that's fruit or bread.

SAUERKRAUT

Because it's often piled onto hot dogs, you may be surprised to learn that sauerkraut is a superfood. Sauerkraut is made from cabbage, which means it has the leafy green's nutritional perks, but thanks to bacteria that break down the natural sugars in the cabbage, sauerkraut is also a fermented food. This fermentation results in a food that's brimming with gut-friendly bacteria (called probiotics) that populate the digestive tract like the probiotics found in yogurt. Consuming foods with good bacteria is beneficial for kids' health because these good bacteria will crowd out the bad bugs that can make kids sick. You can find real sauerkraut in the refrigerated section; make sure it doesn't contain vinegar, sugar, or other additives (the simplest are just cabbage and salt).

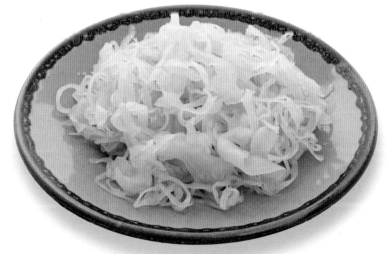

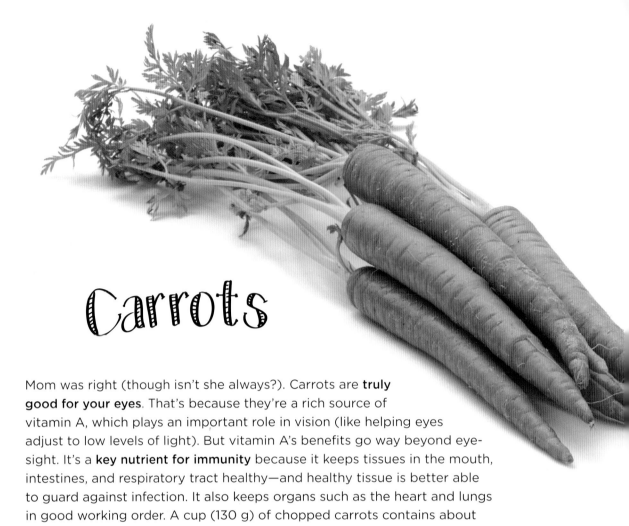

Carrots

Mom was right (though isn't she always?). Carrots are **truly good for your eyes**. That's because they're a rich source of vitamin A, which plays an important role in vision (like helping eyes adjust to low levels of light). But vitamin A's benefits go way beyond eyesight. It's a **key nutrient for immunity** because it keeps tissues in the mouth, intestines, and respiratory tract healthy—and healthy tissue is better able to guard against infection. It also keeps organs such as the heart and lungs in good working order. A cup (130 g) of chopped carrots contains about three grams of fiber and is a good source of magnesium, which **helps build healthy bones**.

Carrots are one of the richest sources of disease-fighting carotenoids, the plant pigments that lend red, yellow, and orange hues to all kinds of produce and convert to vitamin A in the body. In fact, carrots pack in more than three times as much as cantaloupe or mangoes. Orange carrots contain a carotenoid called beta-carotene. (Fun fact: Eating a lot of foods rich in beta-carotene, which gives carrots their color, can temporarily tint your skin!) Substances in carrots such as polyphenols and vitamins also work as antioxidants. Antioxidants are powerful because they neutralize free radicals, which are atoms or groups of atoms that travel around the body and cause damage to cells.

Though orange is the most common, you're likely seeing carrots of other colors on shelves too. If you spot a "rainbow" carrot mix at your store, snag it. It offers a variety of shades including white, red, purple, yellow, and orange—and the bright colors (and fun name) may encourage kids to dig in. Each color contains a different compound with different health benefits. Lutein in yellow carrots is good for vision, lycopene in red carrots may have anticancer properties, and anthocyanins in purple carrots may help protect the heart.

Sweet Carrot Salad

I first ate shredded carrot salad as a high school exchange student in France, where it's a standby starter—especially for children. This simple salad is a fun and novel way to serve carrots, tossed with a sweet dressing and studded with pomegranate seeds.

2 tablespoons (30 ml) fresh orange juice (or bottled OJ)
1 tablespoon (20 g) honey
1 teaspoon apple cider vinegar
⅛ teaspoon salt
2 cups (220 g) shredded carrots
¼ cup (43 g) pomegranate seeds (optional)

In a small bowl, mix together the orange juice, honey, vinegar, and salt. Add the carrots and toss well. Portion into 4 small bowls and top with pomegranate seeds, if desired. If making ahead, keep the carrots and dressing separate until ready to serve.

Yield: 4 servings

✳ "TRY IT" TIP

Sounds crazy, but simply cutting veggies in a different shape or serving them in different sizes can make a big difference. If your kids refuse baby carrots, they might like carrot "coins" with dip. My younger son used to love when I served him a large carrot with the greens so he could eat it "like a rabbit." (Bonus: I sometimes find that whole carrots are sweeter than bagged baby carrots.)

Good to Know

Despite internet rumors, baby carrots are not soaked in harmful chemicals during processing. It's true that they're washed in a solution that contains chlorine, but the levels are similar to what you'd find in regular tap water.

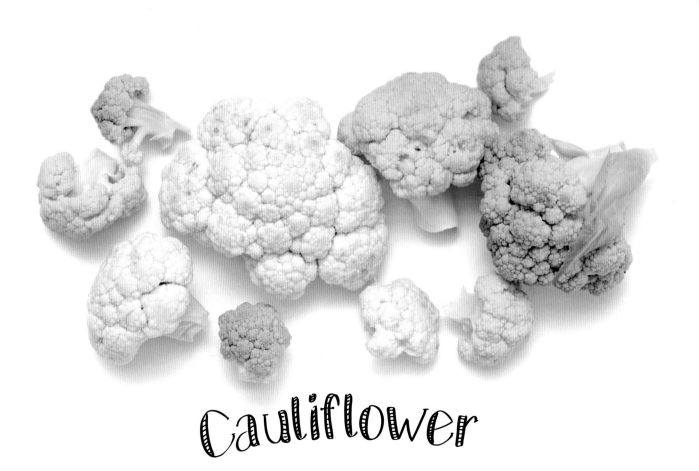

Cauliflower

Talk about trendy! The once forgotten filler on veggie trays has staged a serious comeback. Thanks to so many people going low carb and gluten free, cauliflower is being mashed like potatoes, pressed into pizza crusts, and pulsed into bits as a stand-in for rice. Thick slices of it are even being grilled and called steaks.

Though white veggies such as cauliflower are sometimes accused of being less nutritious than their colorful counterparts, we now know that pale produce still packs a wallop too. Cauliflower is **rich in nutrients such as vitamin C and fiber**, plus **potassium and folate**. And like its cruciferous cousins broccoli and cabbage, cauliflower contains natural plant compounds that may **help the body combat cancerous cells** (those same ones that broccoli has that give off an odor while cooking).

In the produce aisles, you'll find heads and florets of cauliflower as well as bags of riced cauliflower already finely chopped (you'll also spot bags of florets, riced, and mashed with the frozen veggies too). If you really want to surprise your kid, check to see if your store carries green or purple varieties. Eat cauliflower raw or steamed, or roast it to bring out its natural sweetness—but avoid boiling it for long periods of time, which zaps the folate content.

Cauliflower Nuggets

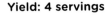

I've never met a kid who didn't like crunchy, dippable finger foods. Serve these nuggets alongside a dish of marinara sauce or ketchup and let them dunk away.

2 cups (240 g) bite-sized cauliflower florets
2 teaspoons olive oil
1 tablespoon (8 g) whole wheat or all-purpose flour
3 tablespoons (21 g) seasoned breadcrumbs
1 tablespoon (5 g) grated Parmesan cheese
½ teaspoon garlic powder
¼ teaspoon salt
¼ teaspoon ground black pepper
1 egg

Preheat the oven to 400°F (200°C) and line a baking sheet with parchment paper or aluminum foil. Rinse and pat the cauliflower dry. In a medium bowl, toss the cauliflower with the olive oil, then sprinkle with the flour and toss until coated. In a small bowl, combine the breadcrumbs, cheese, garlic powder, salt, and pepper. In another bowl, beat the egg. Dip the florets into the egg and then dredge in the breadcrumb mixture, turning to coat. Place the florets on the baking sheet and bake for 20 minutes, gently turning the florets with tongs halfway through the cooking time.

Yield: 4 servings

 "TRY IT" TIP

Go slow with picky eaters. Instead of serving straight-up mashed cauliflower, steam and mash a small amount along with regular mashed potatoes. As they get used to the taste and texture, slowly tweak the ratio to incorporate more cauliflower.

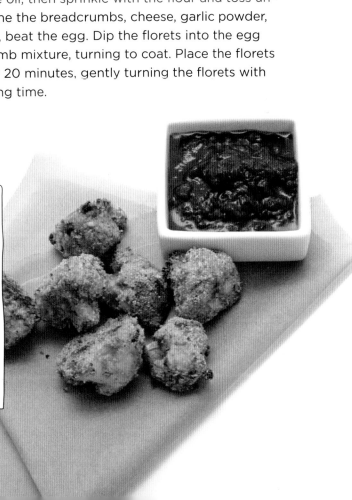

Celery

Celery is often dismissed as low-cal, nutritionally lame diet food. But celery actually contains a respectable amount of **vitamin C and folate** (a B vitamin) plus **a little bit of fiber**. It's packed with water, so it's **hydrating and refreshing**. And if your kids like their veggies extra crunchy, it's a perfect choice.

The bunch of celery, called a stalk, is made up of individual celery "ribs." Bright green ribs have slightly more vitamins, though the lighter green ones may be more flavorful. Be sure the stalks are rigid and look crisp (not limp) when you buy them. Celery will easily freeze, so keep it away from the back of the fridge, where it's coldest. Remove the ribs and thoroughly rinse before serving because dirt and debris like to hide inside. And if you find that the ribs have become rubbery and wilted, cut them into smaller pieces, submerge them in a container of cold water, and refrigerate. They'll crisp right back up!

You can serve celery as sticks with carrots and a favorite dip. My fourth grader loves munching on them cut crosswise into half-moons, which are also fun tossed into salads. The ribs make a fun vessel for nut butter, cream cheese, or hummus. Also, don't toss the leafy tops. Instead, stash them in a plastic bag in your freezer to flavor future soups and broth.

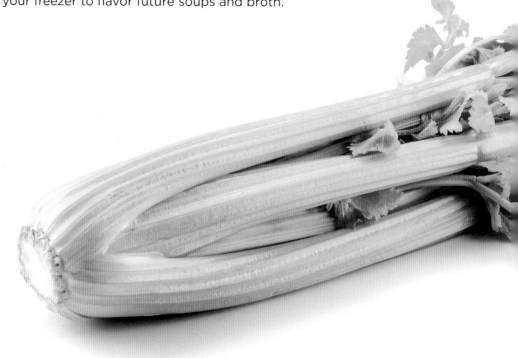

"TRY IT" TIP

If your child is wary of celery, start with the small ribs at the very center of the stalk. They tend to be the most tender and sweet. If your child doesn't like the stringy texture of the outer ribs, simply remove the tough parts with a vegetable peeler.

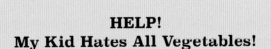

HELP!
My Kid Hates All Vegetables!

Deep, cleansing breaths. This can be frustrating for sure, but it's important to stay calm. Pressuring (or even forcing) a child to take bites of something he doesn't want can make him be even more resistant. Keep offering vegetables in different ways, serve them at most meals, model good habits by eating plenty of veggies yourself, and be patient. In the meantime, keep in mind that if your child eats fruit, he's likely getting a lot of the same nutrients he would nab in vegetables, such as vitamin C, vitamin A, folate, and potassium.

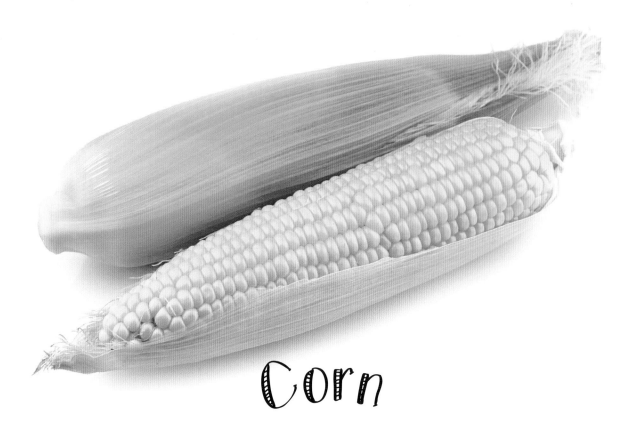

Corn

As a veggie, corn ranks as a favorite among kids—but it's also a bit misunderstood. Corn is a starchy vegetable, which means it has more carbohydrates than its non-starchy counterparts such as broccoli or spinach, which has given corn a bad name in some circles. Some people think corn is nutritionally weak or contains too much sugar. But the reality is, a half-cup (83 g), kid-sized portion contains potassium, magnesium, B vitamins, and vitamin C. And a medium ear of corn has just one-third of the natural sugar of a medium apple. (Fun fact: The average ear of corn has 800 kernels!)

Corn is also a good source of fiber, especially insoluble fiber that can help keep kids regular. And yes, your child might spy some corn kernels in her poop. That's because the body can't fully digest the outer coatings of the kernels. If you buy whole ears of corn in the husk, keep them intact until you're ready to eat them (if they're already husked, store them in a plastic bag to keep them fresh). Corn is sweetest when it's eaten soon after it's picked. But frozen corn, which is typically processed soon after harvest, is a healthy choice too.

As a cereal grain, corn is the most widely produced grain in the world (where it's usually called maize). Naturally gluten free, the grain is rich in vitamin A and antioxidants. Look for "whole grain corn" on the label when buying cereal, cornmeal, or other foods such as grits and polenta.

Brown Bag Popcorn

Store-bought microwave popcorn's got nothing on the homemade kind. Who knew it was this easy to DIY? All you need is popcorn, oil, and a simple brown paper bag. Even better: Popcorn is a natural whole grain!

¼ cup (65 g) popcorn kernels
1 teaspoon vegetable or canola oil

Mix the kernels and oil in a small bowl. Pour into a paper lunch bag and fold down the top twice. Microwave on high power for 1 to 2 minutes, stopping when the popping slows way down or stops. Pour into a bowl and sprinkle with a bit of salt, Parmesan cheese, or other toppings, as desired.

Yield: About 5 cups

Good to Know

Popcorn is a natural whole grain that's also rich in fiber. In a study published in the *Journal of the American Dietetic Association,* kids and adults who regularly ate popcorn took in 250 percent more whole grains and 22 percent more fiber than people who didn't munch on it.

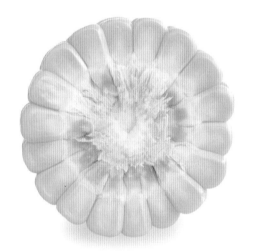

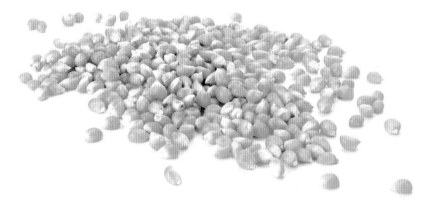

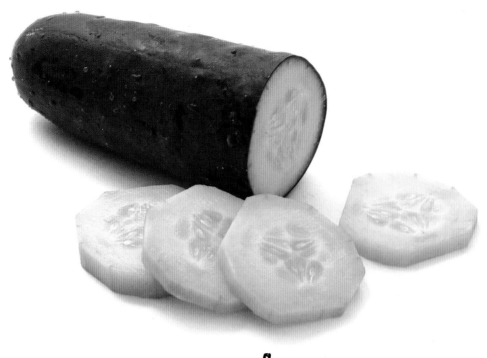

Cucumbers

I'll be honest: This summer veggie (technically a fruit!) is not exactly packed with nutrients. Cucumbers contain some vitamin K, which helps blood clot normally, and some potassium, which helps regulate blood pressure. But your child would need to eat an awful lot of cucumbers to nab meaningful amounts. There may also be a **wee bit of antioxidant power** packed into each cuke, but clearly your kids would get more bang for their buck eating other veggies and fruit. So why am I including them here? What cucumbers *do* have going for them is a very high water content—they're 96 percent water!—which makes them **filling and low in calories**. That's exactly the kind of food that's helpful to love as kids grow into adults. Diets rich in filling, low-calorie veggies can help kids and grown-ups maintain a healthy weight. That high water content also makes cukes refreshing and counts toward your child's daily fluid needs, which is especially helpful during the summer with high temperatures and plenty of sweaty outdoor play.

When buying cucumbers, look for ones with dark green skin (never yellow). They'll last about a week in the crisper drawer. If your kids don't love the seeds, you can slice it lengthwise and scoop them out using a spoon. Then slice the halves into cucumber "moons" to toss onto salads. When I was growing up, my mom made a simple cucumber salad all summer long from garden cukes: sliced cucumbers dressed in apple cider vinegar or rice vinegar mixed with a drizzle of water and sprinkled with salt and pepper.

And if your kid already likes pickles, you may want to inform her that pickles are actually cucumbers. While pickles are typically high in sodium, those packed in a saltwater brine (not vinegar) are usually a **good source of probiotics,** friendly bacteria good for your child's gut.

Good to Know

Picky eating is a normal part of child development, starting in the toddler years and typically improving when kids reach school age. But some kids' habits go above and beyond what's considered standard-issue finicky eating. Here are some red flags that your child may need some help with her eating:

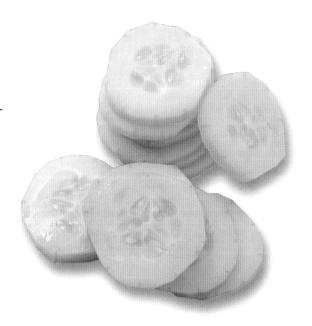

- Eating fewer than 20 foods
- Experiencing weight loss or slow growth
- Refusing to eat for long periods of time
- Acting afraid or angry at mealtime

If this sounds like your child, talk to your pediatrician about getting a referral to someone who specializes in children's eating (and see the resources section at the end of this book for help too).

✳ "TRY IT" TIP

Talk up how delicious healthy foods taste. In one study published in the *Journal of Consumer Research,* scientists read two versions of a story to preschoolers about a girl eating crackers. One version described the crackers as making the girl healthy and strong. The other version described the crackers as being yummy. When the kids were given crackers after hearing the story, the ones who heard the version about "healthy" crackers ate fewer than the other group and rated them as being less tasty.

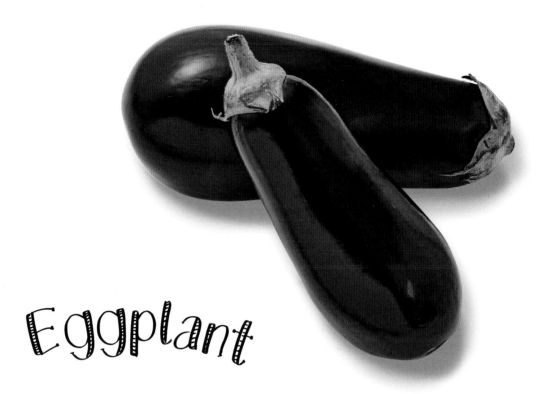

Eggplant

If you're a parent of an adventurous eater, you probably think eggplant is no big deal. (Lucky you!) But if you've got a picky eater, you're likely wondering why I'm including eggplant in this book when your kids won't even touch carrots. Believe me though, every veggie is worth a try. You never know what your kid is going to like—so stay with me!

Like potatoes, the eggplant is a member of the nightshade family. It grows on a vine like tomatoes and comes in different sizes and shapes, from long, thin Japanese eggplant to fat, pear-shaped Italian eggplant. When shopping, look for eggplants that look shiny and avoid any with wrinkled skin (and be gentle with them because they bruise easily).

The eggplant isn't a powerhouse of vitamins and minerals, though it has some **potassium and magnesium**, plus **fiber that helps make it filling**. But like many other veggies, the true health perks of eggplant are in the **beneficial plant compounds**, many of which are pigments found in the skin (or just under the skin). Not only do these pigments give eggplant its deep purple color, but they also work like free-radical scavengers in the body. While the skin has the highest content of these beneficial compounds, they're found throughout the vegetable, so it's okay to peel off the skin if that might be a deal breaker for getting your child to try it. Also, just like with asparagus, the antioxidant content and power intensify when the eggplant is cooked.

Eggplant contains a lot of moisture, so to keep it from becoming soggy and unappetizing when cooked, pull out some of the moisture before cooking. To do this, cut the eggplant in whatever shape you want (such as rounds, slices, or cubes), then generously sprinkle it with salt and let it sit for at least

30 minutes in a colander. Before cooking, rinse off the salt and dry the eggplant, removing even more moisture by pressing it with a paper towel or clean kitchen towel. Salting it this way can also reduce some of the natural bitterness. If your kids are still wary of the spongy texture, try cutting it into small cubes and roasting it. The center gets soft and creamy, but the edges stay crispy, similar to roasted potatoes.

Q: Are Veggie Chips a Healthy Snack?

Read ingredient lists carefully on packaged veggie chips and "straws." Most are made with potato flour, coloring, and flavoring—and possibly some veggie purée. So they're hardly a one-for-one swap for real veggies. A little closer to the real deal are dehydrated veggies (sometimes found in the bulk section of grocery stores), which are a fun and crunchy way to get kids more comfortable with veggies such as green beans, peas, and carrots.

✳ "TRY IT" TIP

Already have hummus fans in your house? Introduce them to baba ghanoush: cooked eggplant puréed with lemon juice, olive oil, and garlic. Serve it with crunchy pita chips and baby carrots.

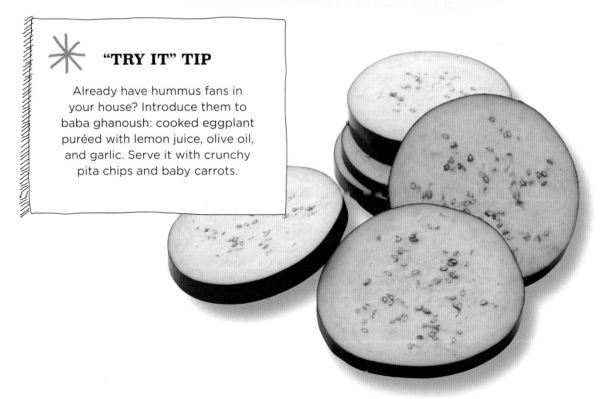

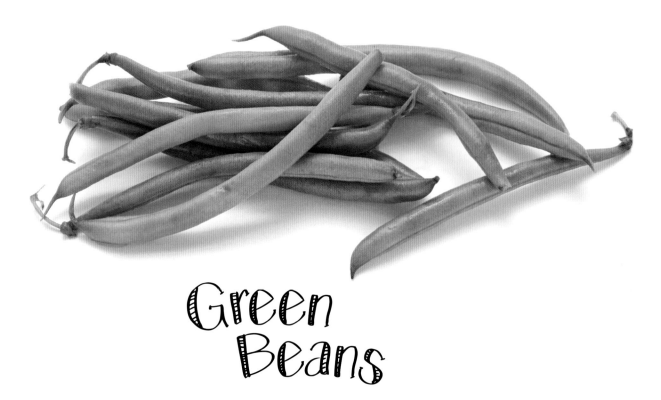

Green Beans

They're not flashy or exotic, but green beans are a reliable side dish and a veggie your kids probably know and just might like. You might have grown up calling them string beans because they used to have a fibrous string running up the side that was removed before eating. Today's beans are stringless thanks to plant engineering. Green snap beans are just one kind of edible-pod bean. You may also spot skinny French beans (haricots verts) and Italian beans at the store.

One major perk of green beans is their fiber content. One cup (100 g) of fresh green beans has **four grams of fiber** (that's a lot, considering that young kids need about twenty grams a day). Beans also contain some potassium, **vitamins A and C for immunity**, vitamin K, and even **a little bit of calcium**.

Be sure not to overcook green beans. Their bright color will fade to an unappealing gray-green. Instead, aim for bright green "al dente" beans, which will still be a little bit firm. You can achieve that by steaming, lightly sautéing, stir-frying (cut beans in half or thirds to make them bite-sized), or blanching. To blanch, drop a few beans at a time into a pot of boiling water and let them cook for 2 to 3 minutes max. You can also roast green beans by tossing them in olive oil and baking at 400°F (200°C) until browned. Or your kids can simply munch on them raw, straight out of the fridge (that's how my younger son likes them!).

Green beans are the third most commonly grown veggie in gardens in the United States (behind tomatoes and peppers). Planting a little patch may encourage your kid to try and like them, and that really goes for any fruit or veggie. When kids are invested in planting, watering, and caring for plants, they're more likely to eat the fruits of their labors. And nothing beats a fresh veggie or fruit warmed by the sun, picked right off the plant.

Q: Are Fresh Vegetables Healthier Than Canned and Frozen?

Not necessarily. In fact, sometimes canned and frozen come out on top. For some veggies, processing enhances healthy compounds—such as the antioxidant lycopene, which becomes even more concentrated after tomatoes are processed. Another perk: Canned and frozen veggies are usually picked mere hours before processing, so there's less time for vitamin loss compared to fresh veggies, which can travel hundreds of miles and spend time sitting on shelves. Perhaps even more importantly, canned and frozen veggies are affordable and convenient, so you can always have them on hand (which means you may eat them more often). When choosing canned veggies, look for sodium-free versions or rinse them before using to remove some of the sodium. For frozen veggies, opt for plain varieties and season them yourself instead of buying ones packed with heavy sauces.

Good to Know

Before using canned vegetables, rinse them under cool water. Rinsing can remove up to a quarter of the added sodium.

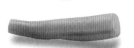

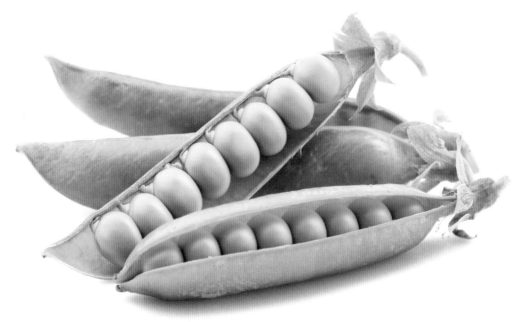

Green Peas

Like corn, green peas are a starchy vegetable, so they're higher in natural sugar than other veggies. But that's okay! They are also **rich in the immune-boosting vitamin A**, and a little half-cup (75 g) serving has three grams of fiber, the same amount in a slice of whole wheat toast. Peas are also a surprising **source of protein**. That half-cup portion has nearly four grams of protein, as much as a half cup of milk. In fact, pea protein is a trendy ingredient right now. It's typically made from yellow peas and added to foods and drinks as a sustainable and healthy way to boost protein content.

Fresh green peas aren't available for very long in the store. But don't write off the frozen variety. They're just as healthy and easy to keep on hand to toss into casseroles, pasta, salads, and even mac and cheese, or serve as an easy side dish. And please don't be afraid to add a little bit of butter and salt. Fat and seasonings can make veggies taste better and encourage your child to try them or eat more of them.

Though they're not as rich in protein, snow peas and sugar snap peas are **good sources of vitamin C** and pack a little bit of fiber and calcium too. Unlike regular green peas, both the pod and the peas are edible. The super-sweet flavor of snap peas makes them especially kid-friendly to pack in lunch boxes to munch raw or add to stir-fries (cut in half to make them bite-sized).

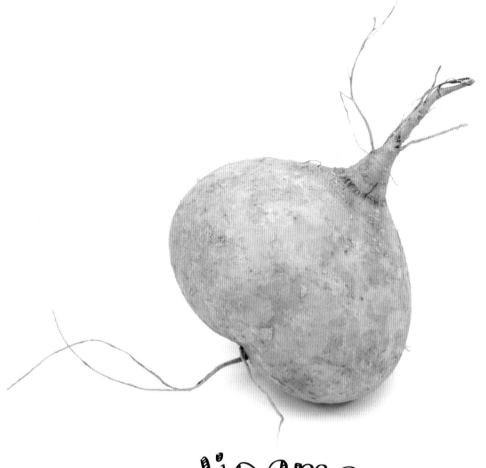

Jicama

If an apple and a potato had a love child, it just might be jicama (pronounced HICK-a-ma). This root veggie, native to Mexico, looks like a cross between a potato and a turnip and tastes vaguely like an apple, but much less sweet. Once you peel away the inedible brown skin with a knife (it's too thick for a vegetable peeler), you can slice up the crisp, white flesh. Jicama is usually eaten raw, sprinkled with lime juice or dunked into dip, or sliced thin for salads and slaws. But you can give it the potato treatment and roast, bake, or boil it too.

Jicama is a **good source of fiber** for fullness and regularity and **magnesium** to help build bone and keep the immune system strong, plus a little bit of potassium and vitamin C. It also contains a fiber called inulin that **acts as a prebiotic**, which means it "feeds" the healthy bacteria in the gut and allows them to flourish. That's important because having a greater number of healthy bacteria can help keep digestion running smoothly and leaves less room for the bad bacteria that can cause illness.

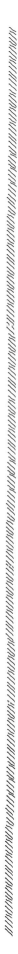

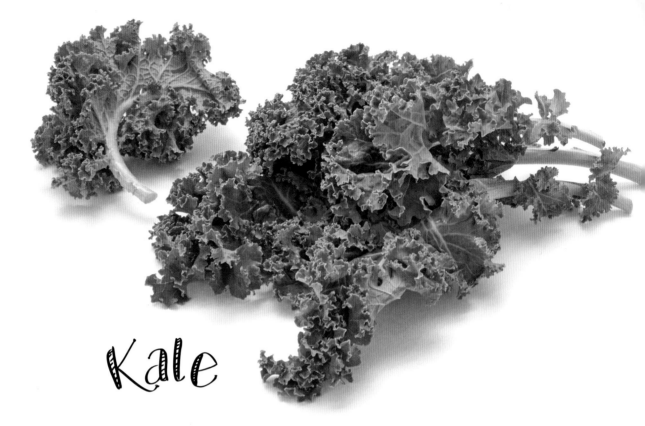

Kale

Contrary to what your Instagram feed is telling you, it is entirely possible to have a healthy diet without eating a pound of kale every day. So if you're not convinced your kid will accept this (admittedly bitter) leafy green, don't despair—but do consider a few tricks that help make kale more kid friendly. First, remove the center stems, which are thick, tough, and unpleasant to chew. To do this, hold the stalk in one hand and use the other to slide along the stem, pulling off the leaves as you go. Second, when you're serving it raw, soften the chewy leaves by "massaging" them with dressing—yes, with your hands (a perfect kitchen task for kids if they're game!).

But yes, kale is worthy of its hype. It contains **iron, potassium, and vitamins A and C** and is a **good source of calcium**. In fact, research published in the *American Journal of Clinical Nutrition* found that the calcium in kale is actually well absorbed by the body—much better than the calcium in other leafy greens such as spinach. Because it's a member of the same family as cauliflower and broccoli, it shows some of the same **anticancer promise** in research too.

When shopping for kale, you'll spot two kinds: lacinato and curly. Lacinato (or "dino") kale is ideal for salads, while curly kale makes for prettier, crunchier chips (see recipe). You can use kale in many recipes that call for other leafy greens, such as soups, egg dishes, and casseroles. You can also put kale into green smoothies, but be warned that it does have a strong flavor, so go easy (or go halfsies with milder-tasting spinach).

Crunchy Kale Chips

Even salad-phobic kids might like munching on these crunchy greens. My younger son calls these addictive!

½ bunch curly kale (about 7 stems' worth)
1½ tablespoons (23 ml) olive oil
Pinch of salt

Preheat the oven to 275°F (140°C). Line a baking sheet with parchment paper.

Pull the kale leaves away from the tough center stems and discard the stems. Tear the leaves into pieces about the size of potato chips. Rinse the leaves and pat dry with a paper towel.

Place the kale in a bowl and drizzle with the olive oil, massaging with your hands to work the oil into the leaves. Sprinkle on the salt and massage again with your hands. Spread the leaves on the baking sheet. Bake for 20 minutes, or until crisp, giving the leaves a stir halfway through. Serve immediately.

Yield: 4 servings

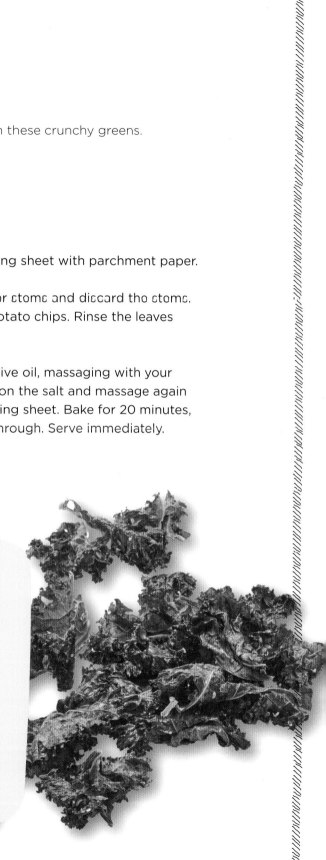

Q: Should We Impose a "Just One Bite" Rule?

Sure, if your child responds well to this dinner table policy. But if your rule is met with resistance, back off. A "one bite" rule can encourage some kids to try new foods (and discover new favorites). For other kids, it turns into a battle of wills—and food shouldn't be a source of conflict at the table. A better route to take for a more resistant crowd: Gently encourage them to take a taste (or serve them a bite on a small, separate dish if that's less threatening), but don't force it.

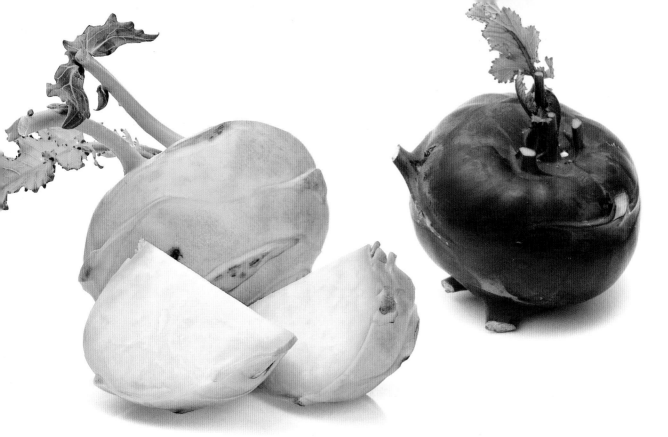

Kohlrabi

Rumor has it that kohlrabi is poised to be the next trendy veggie, which means that, for once in my life, I'm actually ahead of a trend! I grew up crunching on this veggie from my father's vegetable garden, and now my kids love it too. But kohlrabi is definitely not a familiar vegetable to most. It's got a decidedly alienlike appearance: a wide, fat bulb with long, leafy stems growing off of it. It looks like a root veggie, and you might mistake it for a turnip. But kohlrabi grows above ground and is a cruciferous veggie like broccoli or cabbage.

You'll find kohlrabi in purple and green varieties, but the flesh inside is white and has a mild and even slightly sweet (or sometimes a bit peppery) flavor, with a texture like a radish. The very thick, tough skin must be peeled away with a paring knife (it's not a job for a flimsy vegetable peeler), and you can slice the flesh into sticks and serve it raw. That's how we like it, sprinkled with salt. Or you can cut it into cubes or slices, toss it with oil, and roast it. Kohlrabi is a **good source of fiber and potassium** for kids (two nutrients they need more of!) and an excellent source of **immune-boosting vitamin C**. Just a half cup (68 g) meets their daily needs.

Mushrooms

Okay, they're not technically a vegetable, but for the sake of convenience (and in the absence of a "Fungi" chapter in this book), we're grouping them into the veggie category. Mushrooms boast some of the same nutrients as vegetables, such as potassium. But unlike veggies, mushrooms have the unique ability to hit the fifth taste sense called umami, a savory and slightly meaty flavor.

Mushrooms also have the distinction of being the only produce that's a **natural source of vitamin D**, a nutrient both kids and grown-ups don't get enough of. Kids in particular need plenty of D to help their bodies soak up bone-building calcium. Like people, mushrooms can actually produce vitamin D with exposure to UV rays. So while mushrooms naturally contain D, some growers are now boosting the vitamin content in their crops even further using UV light treatment. White button and brown cremini mushrooms (sometimes labeled "baby bellas") are the varieties most likely to have the boosted D, but check the Nutrition Facts panel on the package to be sure.

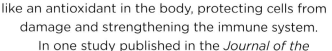

Mushrooms are also a **good source of selenium**, a mineral that acts like an antioxidant in the body, protecting cells from damage and strengthening the immune system. In one study published in the *Journal of the American College of Nutrition,* adults who ate mushrooms every day for a month had immune cells that were stronger and quicker to react to invaders such as viruses and bacteria. Though your kid probably isn't going to eat mushrooms every day, it's good to know that baking them onto pizza or tossing them into stir-fries might be boosting his health even a little bit.

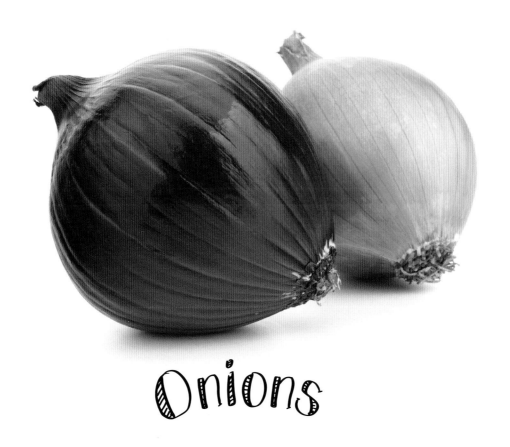

Onions

"Why is it that my children can't find their shoes but can locate a tiny speck of onion in their dinner?" So goes a widely circulated Facebook meme—popular because so many parents can relate. I'll admit I was one of those kids too, removing bits of onion from my spaghetti sauce with surgical precision. I'm happy to report that I grew out of it (and your kids likely will too). But in the meantime, if you've got an onion-phobic brood, try my trick: I finely chop onions in the food processor, almost to a purée, before adding them to a dish. To save time, I process several at once and stash portions in the freezer in small zip-top bags. When a recipe calls for some chopped onion, I have some on hand to toss in!

But whatever you do, don't take onions out of circulation. Not only are they an effective and **sodium-free way to add flavor** to recipes, but they're also jam-packed with health benefits. A member of the allium family that includes garlic and shallots, onions contain a few different substances that protect health. They have sulfur-containing compounds (the same ones that make onions so fragrant) that may **help lower the risk for certain kinds of cancers** and quercetin, an antioxidant that may **help lower blood pressure**. Red and yellow onions contain anthocyanins, the pigments that give them their color and work as antioxidants too. Onions also have a little bit of potassium, calcium, fiber, and folate.

Store whole onions in a cool, dry place (not the refrigerator)—and not in a plastic bag or alongside potatoes, both of which can cause them to spoil. Once cut, wrap them tightly or place in a container and refrigerate. If your kids hightail it out of the kitchen when you're slicing onions (like mine do), that's because cut onions release a gas that irritates the eyes. You might be able to reduce the tears by saving the root end to cut last, because it's more concentrated with the tear-producing compound. Chilling the onion before cutting it or slicing it while it's submerged in water might help too.

Good to Know

Onions contain fructans, which are carbohydrates that work as prebiotics for the healthy bacteria (called probiotics) to feed on in the digestive system. These are good for gut health, but fructans can cause GI upset such as gas and bloating for some sensitive people, especially those who have irritable bowel syndrome.

Q: Does My Child Need to Take a Multivitamin?

No, as long as she eats a fairy balanced diet and a variety of foods. But if your child is a very picky eater, eating few to no fruits and vegetables and limited numbers of other foods, a multivitamin is a helpful insurance policy. Specific vitamins and minerals may make sense for some kids: For instance, children who are low in iron may need to take a supplement. And most kids benefit from taking 400 IU of vitamin D a day. Talk to your child's pediatrician or dietitian about supplements and remember to buy a children's formulation, avoiding any with very high Daily Values (more than 100 percent).

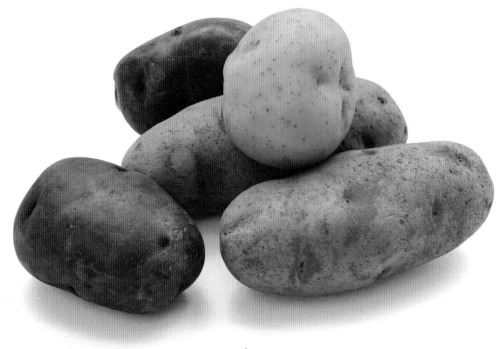

Potatoes

The poor, maligned spud has gotten an awfully bad rep, accused of being too starchy and nutritionally wimpy. But potatoes are a surprisingly respectable nutrient package. They're an **excellent source of vitamin C** (one medium tater meets a kid's daily needs), and vitamin C also helps the body better soak up the iron in potatoes. They're a concentrated source of potassium, even better than bananas. They're also **rich in fiber**, with three grams in a medium spud, found in both the flesh and the skin. In fact, there's a common misconception that peeling potatoes removes all the nutrition, but up to two-thirds of the fiber is actually in the flesh—and most of the other nutrients are located in the flesh too.

More than 200 varieties of potatoes are sold in the United States, and they're all a little bit different. Some have extra-special health-boosting properties. Purple and red potatoes both contain plant chemicals called anthocyanins, which give them their hue. Anthocyanins are a kind of antioxidant, which means they can help guard cells against damage. Another stealth benefit of all potatoes: When they're cooked and cooled (like in potato salad), they're high in something called resistant starch, a carb that resists digestion in the small intestine and is broken down in the large intestine instead. Resistant starch may help kids feel full and **increase the healthy bacteria in the gut**.

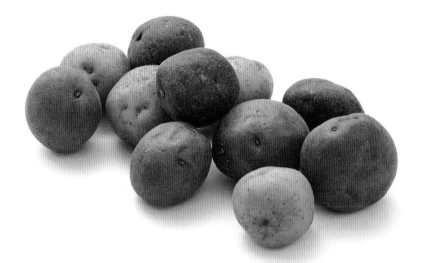

Unfortunately, the most popular form of potatoes is the french fry, which ranks as the most frequently consumed vegetable among toddlers, according to a 2017 study in *Pediatrics*. Though french fries are okay every once in a while, they shouldn't be a staple. In research from the University of Washington, children who ate baked, boiled, and roasted potatoes took in more potassium and vitamin C than those who didn't eat potatoes.

Good to Know

You shouldn't fear salt and fat when it comes to serving veggies. A little pat of butter or a sprinkle of salt can go a long way in giving veggies and other healthy foods extra appeal.

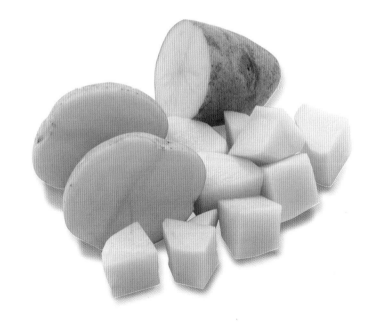

Pumpkin

The obsession with all things pumpkin spice reaches a frenzy in the fall, but pumpkin is so healthy it really should be savored all year long. Thanks to its deep orange color, pumpkin is **loaded with beta-carotene**, a pigment that works to neutralize cell-damaging free radicals. It has sky-high amounts of **immune-boosting vitamin A**—more than 200 percent what you'd need in a day in a little half-cup (58 g) serving!

Keep in mind that regular carving pumpkins aren't good for eating. Instead, you'll want to look for "pie" or "sugar" pumpkins, which are sweeter and not as stringy. To prep one, cut off the stem end, cut the pumpkin in half, and scrape out the seeds and stringy bits. Then place it, skin-side down, in a baking dish with a quarter-inch (6 mm) of water and bake at 350°F (180°C) for 30 to 60 minutes, or until tender. Or you can simply buy canned pumpkin purée (not pumpkin pie filling)—you can't beat the convenience, and it's loaded with nutrition. You can add pumpkin purée to muffins, baked pasta, oatmeal, smoothies, chili, and mac and cheese. (Got extra purée after making a recipe? Freeze it in ice cube trays, then pop the cubes into a freezer bag until you need some.)

Also make sure to keep the pepitas, or pumpkin seeds. They're a valuable part of the pumpkin and too nutritious to toss. Unshelled pumpkin seeds are the kind you scoop out before carving a jack-o'-lantern (you can rinse, dry, and roast them in the oven until crisp!). You can also buy shelled pepitas, which are actually green. Either way, pumpkin seeds are **packed with protein,** with a whopping eight grams in a quarter-cup (16 g) serving, plus iron, potassium, and omega-3 fats. They also contain lignans, a kind of plant chemical that may have anticancer powers.

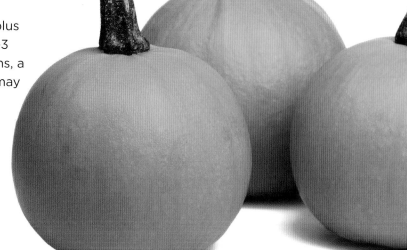

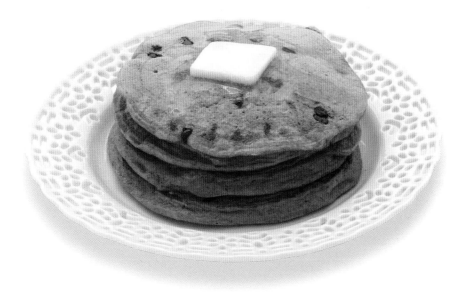

Pumpkin Chocolate Chip Pancakes

Puréed pumpkin gives these hotcakes flavor, color, and a little nutritional boost.

1 cup (230 g) plain whole-milk yogurt
½ cup (124 g) pumpkin purée
¾ cup (90 g) white whole wheat flour
(or regular whole wheat flour)
1 tablespoon (20 g) maple syrup
2 teaspoons baking powder
½ teaspoon vanilla extract
¼ teaspoon salt
¼ teaspoon pumpkin pie spice
¼ teaspoon ground cinnamon
2 eggs, beaten
¼ cup (44 g) mini chocolate chips (or regular if you don't have mini)
Nonstick cooking spray, for preparing the griddle

Good to Know

You can swap pumpkin purée for fats and eggs in a recipe. For every egg in a recipe, use ¼ cup (62 g) pumpkin purée instead. Swap it one for one for butter or oil.

In a bowl, combine the yogurt, pumpkin purée, flour, maple syrup, baking powder, vanilla, salt, pumpkin pie spice, and cinnamon. Add the eggs and stir until combined. Gently fold in the chocolate chips. Using a ¼ cup (60 ml) measuring cup, drop scoops of the batter onto a hot griddle or pan coated with cooking spray. Flip when browned on the bottom and bubbly around the edges.

Yield: 16 pancakes

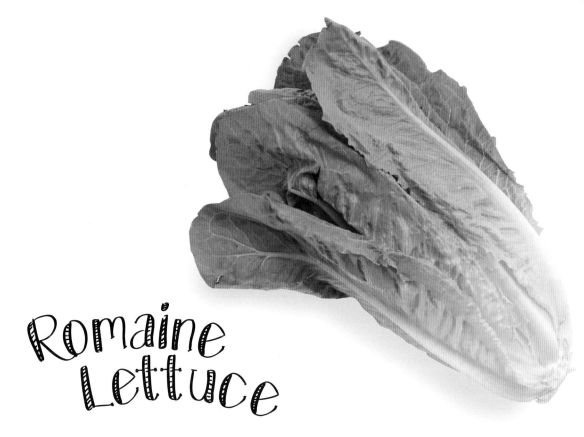

Romaine Lettuce

When my younger son was a dinosaur-obsessed toddler, we played a little game involving lettuce: I would hold leaves out to him, and he would pretend he was an herbivore dino, ambling along on all fours and reaching up to nibble on the lettuce like it was a tree. Years later, he still likes lettuce and will happily munch on plain leaves right off the cutting board. Letting your kids play with food can actually be productive!

Romaine certainly isn't the only lettuce you can feed your kids, and the more greens you can introduce to your kids, the better. There are so many varieties, and they all have slightly different flavors and textures. But romaine is a great starter lettuce for kids because it's mild-tasting and crunchy. It's also a nutritious variety. Compared to iceberg, romaine has four times more **vitamin C and double the calcium** and is loaded with lutein and zeaxanthin, antioxidants that can help **protect the eyes from disease**.

Romaine is the star ingredient of Caesar salad. If your kids already like ranch dressing, they may be open to Caesar too. Look for hearts of romaine, which are the inner, crunchier leaves. It goes without saying, but you're more likely to serve greens if they're already prepped. To prep lettuce for the week, rinse bunches of romaine and dry them in a salad spinner or with a clean towel, then store in plastic bags in the refrigerator. Include a dry paper towel in the bag to absorb any excess moisture, which can lead to decay.

Spinach

As leafy greens go, spinach has a rock-solid reputation for being one of the most nutritious. Its dark green hue comes from plant compounds called carotenoids that are natural disease fighters and health protectors. Two of these carotenoids, lutein and zeaxanthin, gather in the retina, where they help **protect the eyes from damage**, including from blue light emitted by computers and TVs. Spinach is also a **good source of fiber, vitamin K, magnesium, and vitamin A**, and even has a little bit of protein. In a recent analysis by the Centers for Disease Control and Prevention, spinach **ranked in the top five "powerhouse" fruits and vegetables**—ones that pack the most nutrition per calorie.

However, Popeye's promises of bulging muscles after eating spinach were a bit exaggerated. Spinach does contain iron (and calcium), but it also contains a chemical called oxalic acid, which makes it harder for the body to absorb those minerals. Your child will still get iron and calcium from spinach, but you'll want to count on other sources for those nutrients too.

Even if your kids don't like plain cooked spinach as a side dish, they might like it other ways. Buy a box of prewashed baby spinach and toss some with cooked pasta just until wilted to add some color and nutrition, layer it onto lasagna, chop it finely and add to meatballs before shaping, or blend a handful into a morning smoothie. But don't discount frozen spinach: Veggies are frozen soon after picking, so much of the nutrition is locked in. Thaw frozen spinach and layer onto lasagna or into stuffed shells (go light to start) or mix into baked egg casseroles.

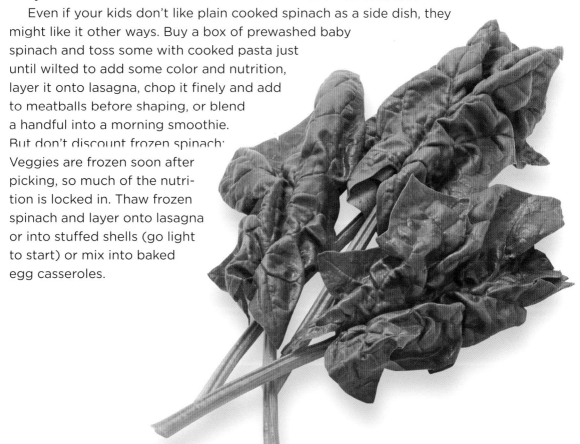

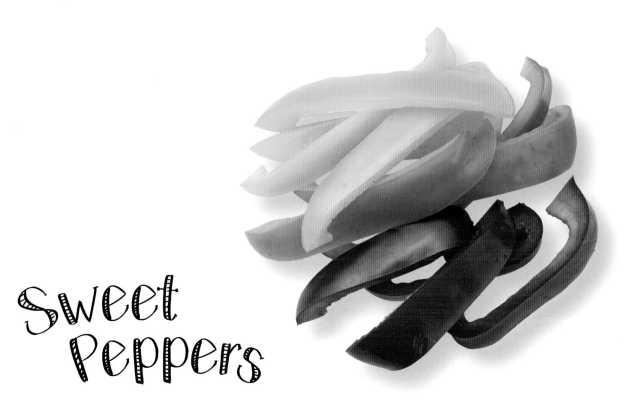

Sweet Peppers

I mean no disrespect to hot peppers. Varieties like chile and jalapeño contain health-protective compounds too, but they're also unquestionably polarizing among the younger set. Some kids embrace heat in their meals, while others (like my youngest) are sensitive to even the briefest shake of black pepper. If your kid likes hot peppers, go for it. Otherwise, you may find more success with the sweet variety. (Fun fact: The spice paprika is made from dried, ground-up bell peppers!)

You'll find sweet peppers in red, orange, yellow, and green. Red is the sweetest, followed by yellow and orange. Green is simply a less ripe version, so it can taste slightly bitter. Though citrus fruits get all the credit for being packed with vitamin C, sweet peppers are no slouch either: A half-cup (75 g) portion of chopped red peppers has more than **double the vitamin C a tween needs in a day**. Besides fortifying the immune system, vitamin C also helps the body better soak up iron from foods. That's especially key when you're serving plant-based sources of iron such as beans and tofu, because that iron isn't as available to the body as the iron from animal foods. Some ideas: Include sweet peppers in a tofu stir-fry or serve raw pepper strips alongside a bean and cheese quesadilla.

Sweet peppers also possess natural plant compounds linked to better health, such as **lycopene in red sweet peppers** that works as an antioxidant, protecting cells from damage and possibly lowering the risk for some cancers (the amount of lycopene is even higher when the peppers are cooked). The carotenoids that give sweet peppers their bright colors also **work as antioxidants**.

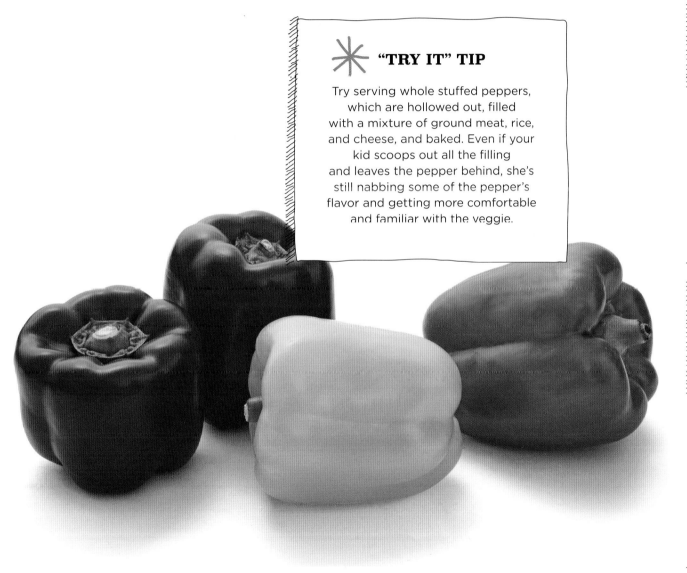

※ **"TRY IT" TIP**

Try serving whole stuffed peppers, which are hollowed out, filled with a mixture of ground meat, rice, and cheese, and baked. Even if your kid scoops out all the filling and leaves the pepper behind, she's still nabbing some of the pepper's flavor and getting more comfortable and familiar with the veggie.

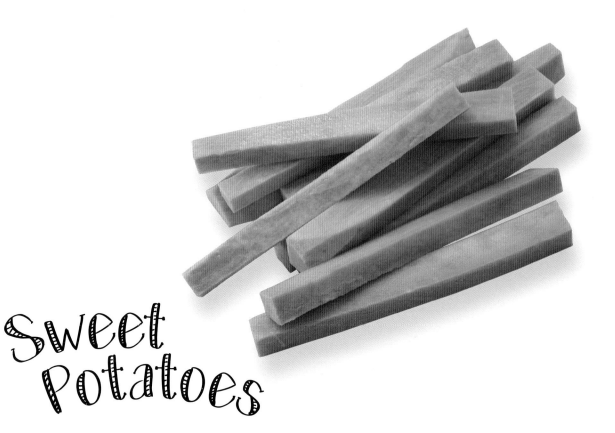

Sweet Potatoes

Crazy but true: Sweet potatoes are actually not related to regular white potatoes. White potatoes are a nightshade, while sweet potatoes are in the morning glory family. And those tubers labeled "yams" in the store? They're not really yams—they're a variety of sweet potatoes. True yams are an African crop that's not typically available in the United States.

Grown by Native Americans long before colonists arrived, sweet potatoes seem decadent because they're naturally sweet—and are often candied and

Q: Do I Need to Buy Organic?

That's the million-dollar question. But there's no one right answer. If you want to avoid chemical pesticides, buying organic is the way to go. But organic also tends to be more expensive—and there's no scientific proof that eating organic is more nutritious than eating conventional or has more health benefits. The most important thing you can do for your child is to serve fruits and vegetables regularly, no matter whether they're conventional or organic. So buy what you can afford, and keep in mind that rinsing produce while rubbing it for 15 to 20 seconds will help remove some of the pesticide residues.

covered in marshmallows for Thanksgiving! But the sweet potato is a healthy pantry staple, with **four grams of fiber** in a one-cup (200 g) serving (that's more than a slice of whole wheat bread contains) and as much potassium as a banana. They're also a rich source of carotenoids such as beta-carotene, the plant pigment that gives their skin and flesh a deep orange color. Beta-carotene converts to vitamin A in the body, a vitamin that's vital for **healthy vision and strong immunity**. Research shows that people who eat a diet high in carotenoid-rich foods (such as sweet potatoes) might have lower rates of certain kinds of cancers.

Though a lot of people think about cooking them in fall and winter, sweet potatoes are available year-round. Keep sweet potatoes in a cool, dry place (not the refrigerator), and then slice them into matchsticks, toss with oil, and bake as "fries" (try them with a sprinkling of cinnamon). Or bake them whole and serve them with a lineup of toppings for a baked potato bar.

Q: Is Real Butter Bad or Good?

For years, butter was nutritional enemy number one, thanks to fears about saturated fat. Some researchers are now questioning whether saturated fat is actually the villain it's portrayed to be, but the most recent Dietary Guidelines for Americans still recommend limiting it. In the meantime, I suggest choosing the fat you like best (whether that's butter or margarine) and using it in moderation—but also incorporating other fats such as olive oil, which is proven in research to be heart healthy.

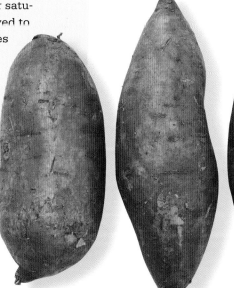

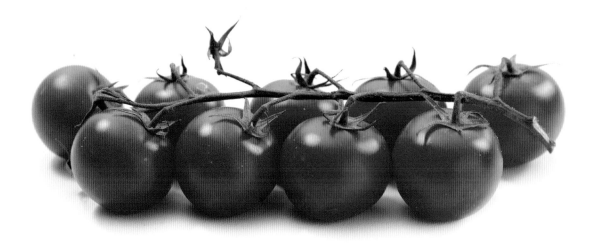

Tomatoes

Yes, tomatoes are technically a fruit, but they're much more likely to be served in a savory green salad rather than a fruit salad. Tomatoes are **rich in potassium**, which has been flagged as a "nutrient of concern" by the government for both kids and grown-ups because most people don't get enough. A half cup (90 g) of chopped tomatoes also has **half the vitamin C young kids need in a day** and is a good source of beta-carotene, a kind of vitamin A.

The pigment that makes tomatoes red is lycopene, and tomatoes account for roughly 85 percent of the lycopene in the American diet. Lycopene has been studied for its potential **power to help lower the risk of cancer**, cardiovascular disease, osteoporosis, and even skin damage caused by UV rays. And here's some welcome news if your kids are hopelessly devoted to ketchup: Lycopene is even better absorbed by the body when tomatoes have been cooked and processed under high heat—as in canned tomatoes, spaghetti sauce, and yes, even your child's beloved ketchup. There's also evidence that consuming lycopene with olive oil may boost absorption too, so drizzle a little bit of olive oil on homemade pizza and use the oil when cooking homemade pasta sauces.

Chopped tomatoes make a sweet first finger food. As your kids get older, they may also like munching on cherry or grape tomatoes. Keep in mind that storing tomatoes in the refrigerator dulls their sweet flavor. They're best kept on the counter, stem-side up.

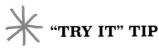

✳ "TRY IT" TIP

Serve veggies when your kids are at their hungriest. I have a house rule of "only veggies in the hour before dinner," and it's been successful at both increasing my kids' veggie intake and ensuring they're hungry when they come to the dinner table. Cherry tomatoes, peppers, and cucumbers are all great choices.

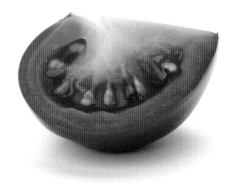

HELP!
My Kid Puts Ketchup on EVERYTHING!

Relax. Those ubiquitous squirts may make you crazy (a perfectly cooked tenderloin *dragged through ketchup?!*). But using ketchup as a familiar dip allows kids to explore new foods safely and comfortably. Though most ketchup is sweetened, remember that some of the sugar is natural from the tomatoes themselves.

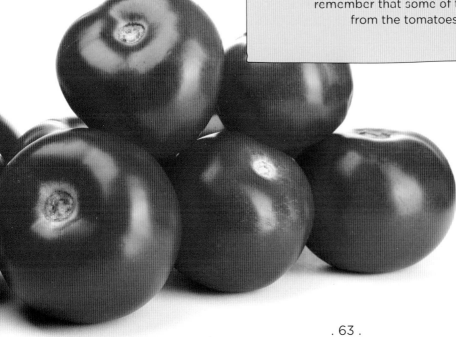

Zucchini

This veggie shot to popularity recently thanks to the nifty kitchen-gadget-of-the-moment, the spiralizer, which turns a regular squash into a bowl of zucchini noodles. And "zoodles" just might be the ticket when it comes to your kids trying and liking zucchini. Let them turn the crank, gobble up the raw spirals straight off the cutting board, or mix them with equal parts cooked spaghetti if they're not sold on eating a whole plate.

Don't have a spiralizer? You can create zucchini "ribbons" with a simple vegetable peeler. Zucchini is also an ideal veggie for kids who are practicing their knife skills, since it's soft and easy to slice. Even shredding zucchini with a box grater or food processor blade and baking it into a loaf of sweet quick bread may help familiarize your child with this veggie—and familiarity is the key to building fondness for a new food! When shopping, look for small, firm zucchini, which are full of flavor and best for eating raw and cooking (the larger ones are better suited for baking).

Though it's lauded as a low-carb replacement for pasta, zucchini offers a whole lot more. This summer squash is **rich in vitamins**, with a cup (120 g) containing nearly all the vitamin C and a third of the vitamin B_6 kids need in a day. It's also a **good source of vitamin K**, which is involved in proper blood clotting, and riboflavin, which helps the body produce energy. It also **packs folate, potassium, and magnesium**.

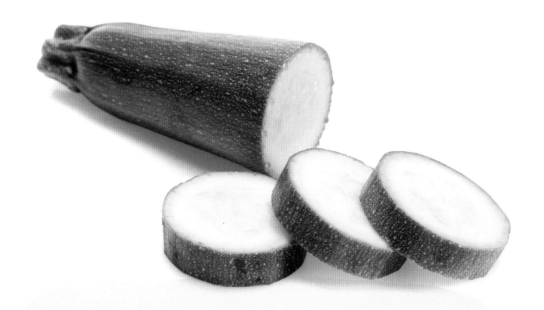

Q: Is it Okay to Sneak Vegetables into Recipes?

Sneaking squash purée into mac and cheese or cooked cauliflower into mashed potatoes has a short-term benefit of getting more nutrients into your child's body. But long term, it won't teach your child any valuable habits (except that Mom and Dad can't be trusted!). If you want to use extra veggies in recipes, don't hide it from your kids. Let them see you whirling black beans into brownies or adding spinach to a smoothie. Keep offering vegetables in their whole form too. It's actually better for your children's lifelong eating habits if they take just one or two bites of vegetables of their own accord than if they eat a whole serving of hidden veggie pasta.

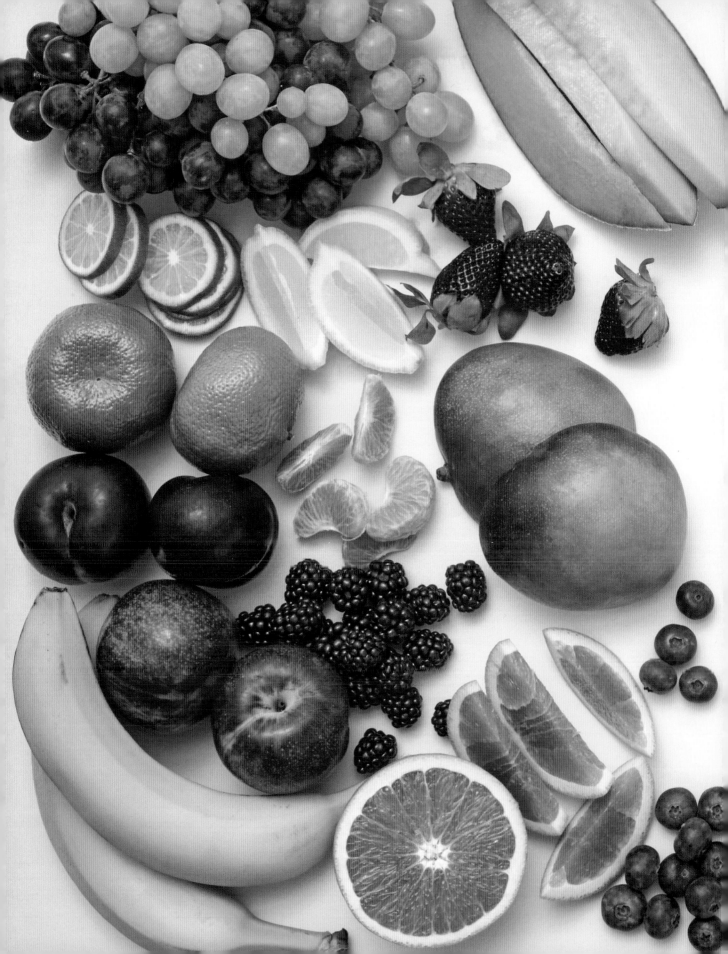

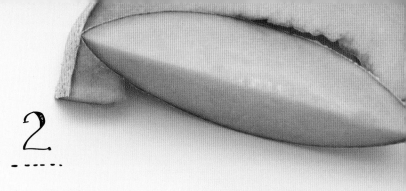

2

Fruits

WHILE MANY PARENTS STRUGGLE TO GET

their kids on board with veggies, "nature's candy" is typically a much easier sell. But it's also easy to fall into a rut—filling the crisper drawer with apples, tossing a banana into lunch bags, and calling it a day. No doubt those fruits deserve their spots in your child's diet, but there are plenty more to explore. Like vegetables, each color of fruit packs slightly different compounds that protect your child's health. So it's smart to offer a wide variety. And fruit's naturally sweet flavor means you're more likely to find success when branching out too.

Though plenty of kids are fans of fruit, only 40 percent get enough each day. Research shows that when kids have more access to fruits (and veggies), they eat more of them. Makes total sense—and even more incentive to make eating fruit easy. Set a bowl of apples and pears within easy reach, toss berries onto cereal in the morning, and pack an extra serving in lunch boxes. Fruit is especially helpful if your child is still learning to like veggies, because so many of vegetables' biggest nutritional perks (such as fiber, vitamins, and minerals) are also found in fruit.

HOW MANY FRUITS DO YOUR KIDS NEED EVERY DAY?

- Ages 2–3: 1 cup*
- Ages 4–8: 1–1$\frac{1}{2}$ cups*
- Ages 9–13: 1$\frac{1}{2}$ cups*
- Ages 14–18: 1$\frac{1}{2}$ cups (girls), 2 cups (boys)*

  Weight varies. Source: United States Department of Agriculture (USDA)

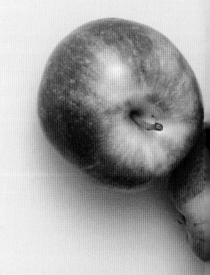

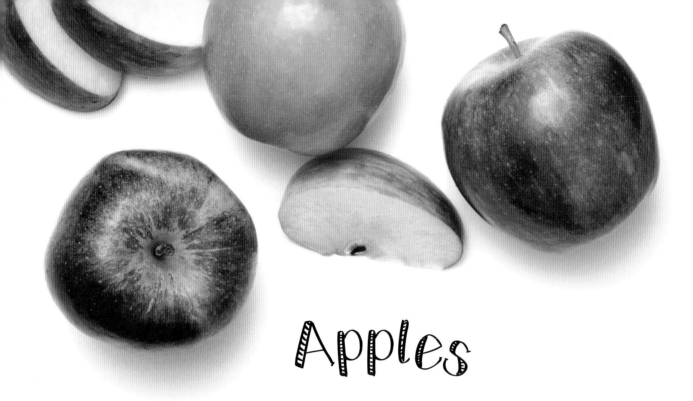

Apples

A no-brainer, right? You probably don't need to convince your kids either: According to a study in *Pediatrics,* apples were ranked as the most frequently eaten fruit for the under-eighteen set. And there's real weight behind the apple-a-day prescription because when your kid crunches into an apple, he's biting into a pretty powerful package. Apples are a **good source of vitamin C**, a vitamin that can help bolster the immune system, and they're high in potassium, a mineral most kids are lacking, which acts like kryptonite to sodium's effects and helps keep blood pressure at a healthy level. Researchers are also studying apples for their potential to fight cancer, asthma, and heart disease. They may even **improve gut health**, because the fruit's pectin (a fiberlike substance) literally feeds the healthy bacteria in the intestines.

If "I'm hungry!" is a familiar refrain at your house, stock up on apples. Thanks to **four grams of fiber** per medium apple and a rich water content, apples rank high on something called the Satiety Index, which rates how filling foods are. Apples even outscore other snacks such as grapes, bananas, crackers, and yogurt. Pair them with a source of protein (such as apple slices dunked in nut butter or served with slices of cheese), and they'll be even more filling.

Because apple varieties are grown year-round, there's no need to think of apples as only a fall fruit. And if your kids aren't crazy about one kind, branch out. Though Red Delicious is one of the most purchased apples, it's not exactly the tastiest. Try other varieties such as Gala, Granny Smith, and Honeycrisp. But whatever you choose, don't peel away the skin—that's where half the fiber and two-thirds of the antioxidant power live!

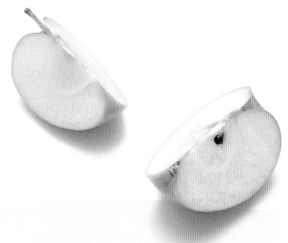

Q: Is Juice Healthy?

Children get about a third of their fruit servings from 100 percent juice. But though most kids love it, it's smart to set limits. Juice is easy to overconsume and delivers a lot of calories and natural sugar—without the beneficial fiber found in the whole fruit. Sipping juice throughout the day also ups the chances of cavities forming and is a common culprit for diarrhea among toddlers. In new guidelines, the American Academy of Pediatrics recommends no juice for babies younger than one year of age and scaled-down portions for older kids: no more than four ounces (120 ml) a day for toddlers, four to six ounces (120 to 175 ml) a day for children ages four to six, and eight ounces (240 ml) for kids ages seven to eighteen.

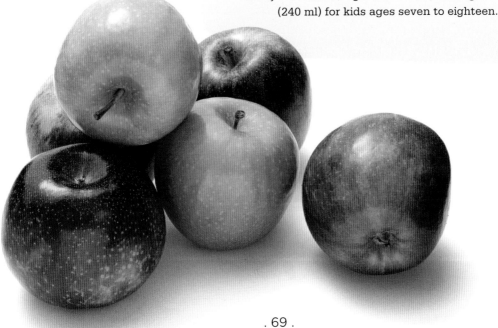

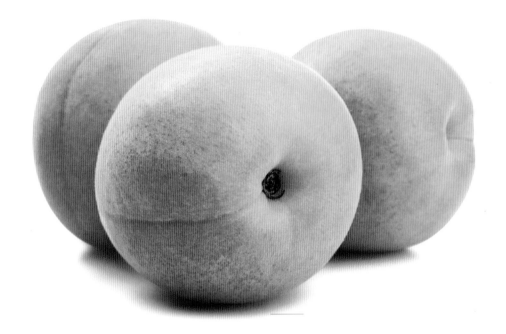

Apricots

Your kids may be more familiar with dried apricots than fresh because most of the crop is sold dried or canned. Fresh apricots have a very short season, another reason some people aren't familiar with them. But grab a bunch when you spot them in early summer. They are the perfect size for little kids and have soft, slightly fuzzy skin and sweet flesh. If the apricots you buy don't give when pressed, let them ripen on the counter for a day or two.

Dried fruits are a concentrated source of nutrients compared to their fresh counterparts, so dried apricots pack more nutrients per serving than fresh. A quarter-cup (33 g) serving of dried apricots is a **good source of iron, vitamin E, vitamin B$_6$, and potassium for kids**. Keep in mind that they may be treated with sulfur dioxide to keep them orange, and that's an additive that can cause stomach upset in some people. You can find untreated dried apricots; they'll just appear slightly brown. Whether fresh, canned, or dried, apricots are also an **excellent source of beta-carotene**, a beneficial plant compound that gives them their orange-pink hue.

Q: How Much Sugar is Too Much for Kids?

According to the Dietary Guidelines for Americans, kids (and adults) should strive for no more than 10 percent of calories from added sugar. Here's what that looks like for kids (ranges are based on calorie needs, which differ depending on body size and activity level):

- Ages 2–3: 6 teaspoons (25 grams) or less

- Ages 4–8: 7–8 teaspoons (28–32 grams) or less

- Ages 9–13: 10–11 teaspoons (40–44 grams) or less

- Ages 14–18: 11–20 teaspoons (44–80 grams) or less

You don't need to obsess over every gram—and there will be days when your child will go way over (and others, way under). But these general ranges are good to keep in mind when comparing products at the store.

Good to Know

Though the package of fruit snacks may say "Made with real fruit!" these little gummies are more like candy than fruit. Many kinds are made with fruit juice concentrate, which is essentially a form of added sugar. Your child doesn't get the same benefits from fruit snacks as he would with fruit. So consider them a sweet treat as you would candy, and stick to real fruit more often.

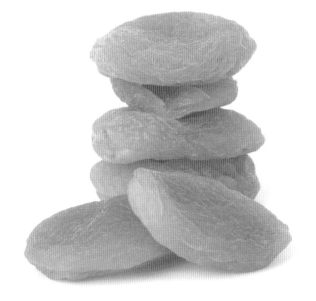

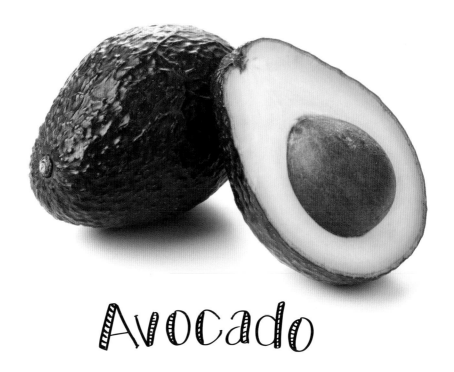

Avocado

When I need to prove the point that "try, try again" should be your motto when it comes to food, I use the avocado as an example. My younger son once cried when I put the tiniest smear of guacamole on his quesadilla. A year later, he was standing at the counter, mashing his own guacamole and scooping up big bites of it with chips. What happened? I just kept offering it and he eventually tried a tiny bite, then another and another. I can't guarantee that will happen with every food you serve, but it gives me hope that my kids can grow to like (and even love) new foods with time. So if your kids don't like avocado yet, keep at it.

Along with having a killer nickname (the "alligator pear"), the avocado has truly unique health benefits among fruit. It's **full of healthy monounsaturated fat**, the kind found in olive oil that's been proven in research to be good for the heart, and it's a **rich source of phytosterols**, a kind of plant chemical that naturally lowers cholesterol levels by blocking some cholesterol from being absorbed by the body. Plus, it is a **good source of potassium** and has a few grams of fiber in each serving (which is about one-third of an avocado).

You'll see avocados in the store in shades of dark or light green and almost black. Some avocados darken as they ripen, but they're best judged by a gentle squeeze. Unripe avocados will be hard to the touch and can take up to five days to ripen on the counter (putting them in a paper bag speeds up the process). Ripe avocados will yield to pressure but won't leave an indentation where you pressed them. If your avocados are ready but you're not, stick them in the fridge, which will slow or stop ripening for a few days. Since cut avocados will turn brown, add some lemon juice to slow down the process. Cover leftover guacamole by pressing plastic wrap directly on the surface. Putting a thin layer of water on top will also prevent browning. Before serving again, just drain the water off and give a good stir.

HOW TO CUT AN AVOCADO

Slice lengthwise around the pit with a knife. Hold one half in each hand and twist in opposite directions to pull the halves apart. Remove the pit with a spoon, then scoop out the flesh with the spoon if you plan to mash it, or gently peel away the skin if you want to slice it.

Starter Guacamole

This is the recipe that got both of my kids happily eating guacamole. Once your kids are on board, take it to the next level by adding diced onion or tomato, salsa, or some chopped fresh cilantro.

2 ripe avocados
Juice of 1 small lime
1 clove garlic, minced or pressed
½ teaspoon salt

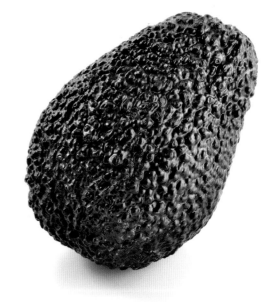

Scoop out the avocado flesh into a bowl. Add the lime juice, garlic, and salt and mash well. Serve with chips or use as a topping for tacos and burritos.

Yield: 6 servings

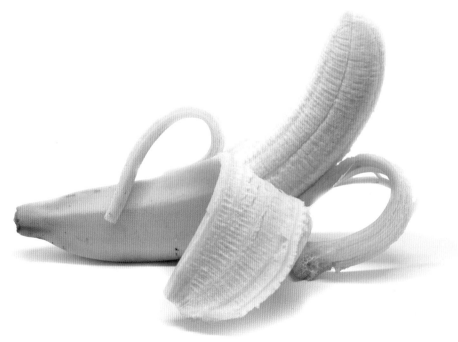

Bananas

There's a good chance that bananas made their first appearance in your child's life on his high chair tray. Soft, sweet, and creamy, they're an ideal first food. And apparently, their luster doesn't wear off, because bananas rank as kids' second favorite fruit, after apples. Cheap, portable, and widely available, bananas are fixtures in countertop fruit bowls and inside lunch boxes for most families.

Potassium is the banana's claim to fame, but truth be told, there are other foods that pack just as much or even more of the mineral, including yogurt, tomato sauce, and orange juice. However, this popular fruit still delivers a nice dose: 422 mg in one medium banana (kids need 3,000 to 4,000 mg per day). Getting enough potassium can stave off muscle cramps and helps regulate fluid balance. The mineral also makes bananas **a worthy recovery food** because they help replenish potassium lost after kids have been sick with vomiting or diarrhea. Plus, the pectin in bananas acts as a binding agent, so the banana is a **cornerstone of the BRAT diet** (along with rice, applesauce, and toast) to treat diarrhea. The fact that they pack some vitamin C makes them an even better snack when fighting or recovering from a bug.

Slightly green and underripe bananas contain something called resistant starch, a carbohydrate that acts like fiber in the body—passing through the small intestine undigested and fermenting in the large intestine, where it can help healthy bacteria flourish. But bananas get softer and sweeter as they ripen and actually have the highest antioxidant levels when they're very ripe (stick them in a bag with an apple to speed ripening). Got an overripe bunch on your counter? Peel and freeze them for future smoothies. Ripe bananas make a creamy, sweet smoothie base, so you might not have to add any sweetener.

➡ Blueberry Banana "Ice Cream"

Prepare to be amazed! Frozen bananas blend up into a dessert that's sweet and creamy like the real deal.

2 bananas, peeled, sliced into chunks, and frozen until firm
½ cup (80 g) frozen blueberries

Place the frozen bananas and blueberries in a food processor or high-speed blender and process or blend, stopping to stir or scrape the sides when needed. The texture will transform from chunky to a smooth, ice cream–like consistency in a matter of minutes. Scoop out and serve.

Yield: 2 servings

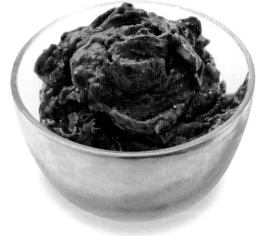

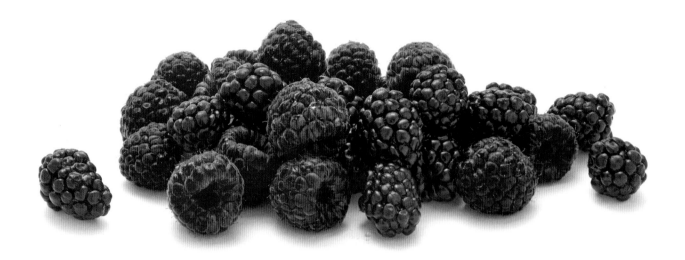

Blackberries & Raspberries

They may be small, but these berries pack a big nutritional perk: They are **some of the highest fiber fruits around**, with about eight grams per cup (about 135 g). That's a third of what kids need in a whole day! Fiber is a nutrient vital to health, not only to keep kids regular but also for heart health, and it's something most kids and adults aren't getting enough of. Both blackberries and raspberries are also **excellent sources of vitamin C**, an antioxidant that fights free radicals in the body and helps fortify the immune system. In fact, when researchers ranked fifty foods on **antioxidant content**, blackberries actually came out on top. Used by Native Americans as food, medicine, and natural dyes, blackberries and raspberries are both rich in plant compounds that are protective to health. For instance, the pigments that make them so colorful, called anthocyanins, are natural disease fighters. Fun fact: The berries are drupelets, which means that, technically, each berry is a cluster of many tiny fruits—each one with its own seed.

If you've ever bought berries only to notice they're moldy when you reach for them, you've found out the hard way that they're extremely fragile (especially red raspberries, which should ideally be eaten within a day or two of purchasing). The berries, which have a short season, tend to be pricey, so it's smart to take steps to prolong their life in your refrigerator. To do this, keep them in the little plastic containers they're packed in, which are designed for storage with venting to allow just the right amount of air in and out. Remove any moldy berries you spy, and rinse berries just before serving. If you snagged a good deal on berries and want to save them for later, rinse them and gently pat dry, spread on a baking sheet in a single layer, freeze until firm, and then transfer them to a freezer bag until you need them. If you buy them already frozen, be sure your bag contains only fruit and no added sugars.

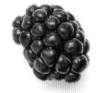

 "TRY IT" TIP

If you like the idea of your child drinking green smoothies—but your kid's not keen on the color—a handful of fresh or frozen blackberries will create a purple shade that might be more pleasing. Just don't hide the spinach from your kids. Show them you're adding it (or make it together) and let them be amazed by how sweet spinach can taste!

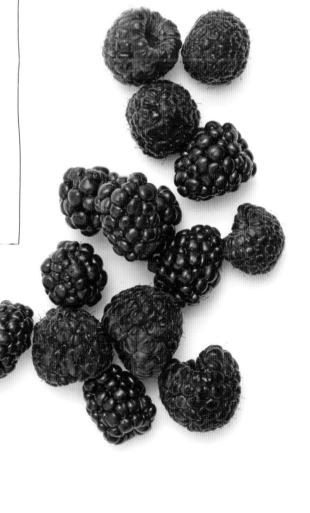

Blueberries

If there really is such a thing as "brain food," blueberries top the list. This small-but-mighty fruit has been studied for its **positive impact on learning and memory** in both adults and kids. Those perks are likely due to the anthocyanins in blueberries—those natural plant chemicals that work as antioxidants in the body and give the berries their blue hue. In fact, blueberries are frequently ranked high for antioxidant capacity compared to other fruits.

Native to North America, blueberries have **all the vitamin C toddlers and preschoolers need** in a day in just one cup (145 g) —plus nearly four grams of fiber. They're also an **excellent source of manganese**, a mineral that's involved in bone development and turning nutrients into energy. Kids can get up to a third of the manganese they need in a day in one cup (145 g) of blueberries.

When buying fresh blueberries, look for firm berries in a deep shade of blue. Don't worry if you see a white, chalky covering on them—that's a natural "bloom" that protects the berries. Avoid any packages with moldy fruit and rinse the berries right before eating. When buying them frozen, the berries should feel loose inside the bag, not clumped together, which indicates they were thawed and refrozen. If you want to freeze your own, rinse them and place them on a baking sheet in a single layer to freeze until solid, then transfer them to a freezer bag.

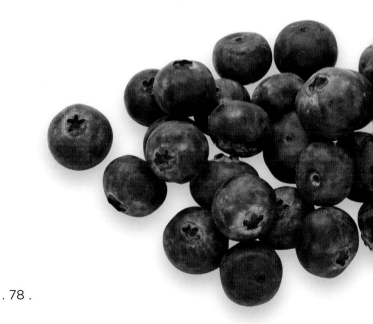

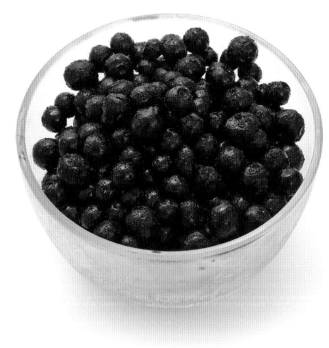

WILD BLUEBERRIES

True to their name, "wild" blueberries grow completely wild. They're darker and more intensely flavored than regular blueberries and have **double the antioxidant power**. Unless you happen to be in Maine during their harvest, you're more likely to find them frozen, not fresh. Look for them in the freezer section of your grocery store along with the rest of the frozen fruit, and snag some to add to smoothies, muffins, and pancakes. In one study published in the *European Journal of Nutrition*, children ages eight to ten scored better on tests for memory and concentration after having a drink made with wild blueberries.

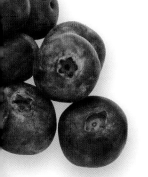

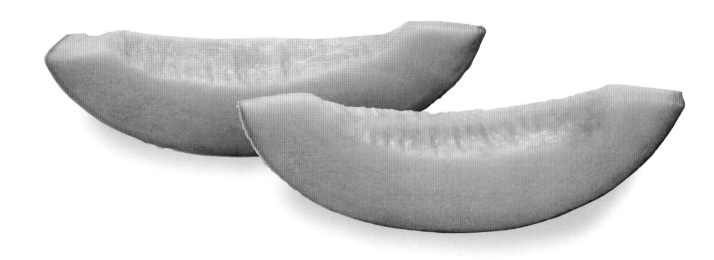

Cantaloupe & Honeydew

It's a shame that so many underripe, tasteless chunks of cantaloupe and honeydew find their way onto fruit trays, giving both melons a bad name. When chosen correctly at the store and eaten at the height of their seasons, cantaloupe and honeydew are nothing short of sweet, juicy summertime perfection.

Cantaloupe, which is technically called a muskmelon, has a sweet-tart flavor, while honeydew is buttery soft and sticky sweet (like honey!). Both are great sources of **vitamin C for building immunity** in kids. A cup (180 g) of cantaloupe or honeydew balls has more than the whole day's worth of C. With its bright orange flesh, cantaloupe has the most beta-carotene of any melon and is rich in vitamin A, another immune-boosting vitamin. Cantaloupe also contains an enzyme that's being studied for its potential as an **antioxidant and anti-inflammatory** in the body (inflammation in the body is thought to be a risk factor for chronic disease). Both melons also have some fiber and are rich in water, so they're **hydrating and refreshing** on a hot day.

When picking a cantaloupe, find one that's heavy for its size and look for yellow or orange skin under the netting (avoid very green skin). The outside of a ripe honeydew should be a creamy yellow-white and waxy, and both should smell fruity at the stem end if they're at room temperature. They won't ripen further once they're off the vine, but keeping them on the counter for a few days may mean they'll be softer and juicier when you slice into them. You'll know they're ready to cut when the stem end "gives" a little bit when pressed (but isn't mushy or spongy). Avoid any melons with very soft or sunken spots.

Good to Know

Always give the outside of cantaloupes a scrub with a produce brush to get into the crevices of the netting, to avoid dragging dirt and bacteria into the flesh when you're slicing it with a knife.

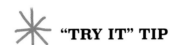

"TRY IT" TIP

Give kids wooden skewers and a bowl of fresh fruit such as melon chunks, strawberries, and grapes so they can build their own fruit kebabs.

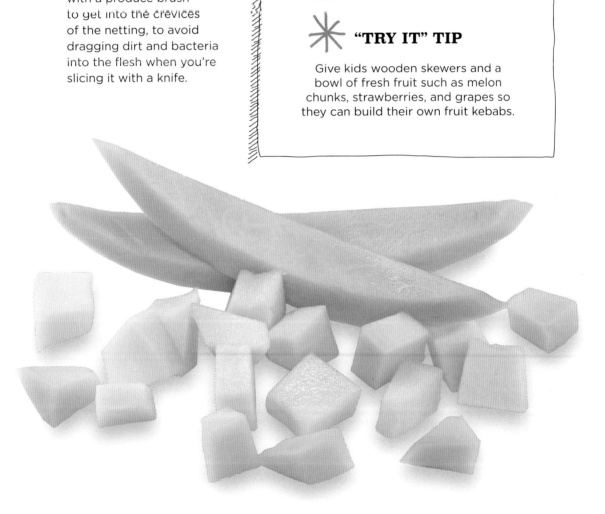

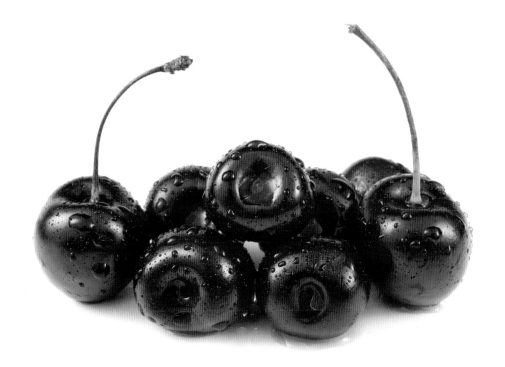

Cherries

Cherry season is short but sweet. While sour cherries are available year-round as prepared pie fillings and sauces, sweet cherries are usually available only from June through August, so get them while you can. Cherries are stone fruits with a pit inside like plums and a good source of potassium for kids. They even deliver a smidge of calcium. A cup (155 g) has about three grams of fiber and half the vitamin C young kids need each day.

Cherries are **rich in antioxidants**, compounds that scavenge cell-damaging free radicals in the body. The plant chemicals that give cherries their brilliant red-purple color, anthocyanins, are found in greater concentration in sweet cherries than sour and have been shown in some animal research to inhibit certain cancers. Cherries also pack quercetin, a particularly potent antioxidant that may **help protect the heart**. The plant chemicals in cherries are also being studied for a possible role in protecting against diabetes as well as inflammation, and that's one reason cherries are being studied for their ability to help reduce muscle soreness and boost recovery after exercise. In fact, some research has found that the anthocyanins in cherries are as effective at **relieving inflammation** as over-the-counter anti-inflammatory meds such as ibuprofen!

When choosing cherries, look for fruit that's plump and firm to the touch. Remove any that are rotting, because (like apples) one bad cherry can spoil the bunch. Your kids might enjoy using a handheld cherry-pitter—or, let's face it, simply spitting out the pits.

Q: Is Dried Fruit Healthy?

People who eat dried fruit have higher-quality diets and healthier body weights, according to government surveys. It's an easy way to get fruit servings when fresh isn't available. But keep a few things in mind: With the exception of raisins and apricots, many kinds of dried fruit are sweetened with added sugar and may even be colored with artificial food dyes. Check labels and, when possible, choose one that contains only fruit. Be aware that some brands may also use sulfur dioxide as a preservative, which can cause stomach upset in some people.

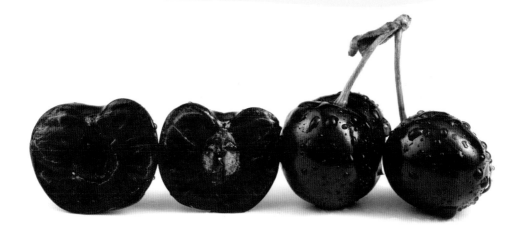

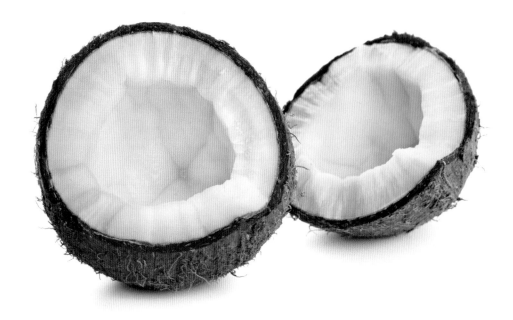

Coconut

Coconut has the distinction of being one of the few fruits that contain fat—namely saturated fat. That may sound like something you'd want to avoid, but here's the scoop: Some of coconut's fatty acids haven't been shown to have a negative effect on cholesterol levels (and may even help boost "good" HDL levels), while others may indeed increase "bad" LDL cholesterol. The net effect could be that coconut has no meaningful effect on cholesterol or heart disease risk either way.

Shredded coconut adds flavor and a light crunch to recipes, along with some **fiber** and a little bit of iron (just look for packages labeled "unsweetened" to avoid added sugar). Coconut water, which is the juice inside the coconut, doesn't contain the coconut's fat. It's considered a sort of **"nature's sports drink"** because it contains some carbohydrate for energy, plus potassium and sodium, two minerals that can be lost through sweat. Coconut milk, made when the meat of the fruit is soaked in water and blended, can be found in cartons and cans. The beverage, sold in cartons, is typically fortified with calcium, vitamin D, and sometimes other nutrients such as magnesium and vitamin A (keep in mind that it's very low in protein and may contain far less calcium than dairy milk). Coconut milk in cans, available in full-fat and lite, lends creaminess and flavor to recipes such as curries and is often used in dairy-free cooking.

A hot pantry staple right now is coconut oil, which can be used as a solid or liquid, depending on the temperature. "Unrefined" or "virgin" coconut oil has a distinct coconut flavor, while "refined" has more of a neutral taste. Though the internet hails coconut oil as a miracle food, research hasn't shown that it lives up to that kind of hype. My advice is to use it when you want the flavor or texture but to continue to use other fats as well, including olive oil, which has been proven to have health benefits.

Q: Is Coconut Sugar Healthy?

Coconut sugar is a trendy sweetener, riding on the coattails of the coconut oil craze. It's made from the sap of coconut palms and has the same number of calories (15) and grams of sugar (4) as a teaspoon of regular table sugar. It's touted as a sweetener that's low on the Glycemic Index (GI), which measures how quickly a food affects your blood sugar after eating it, but that doesn't make it healthy. There are also claims that it's packed with nutrients, but you'd have to eat large amounts of coconut sugar to get meaningful amounts of any nutrient beyond carbohydrates from sugar. Use it in moderation, just like you would any sweetener.

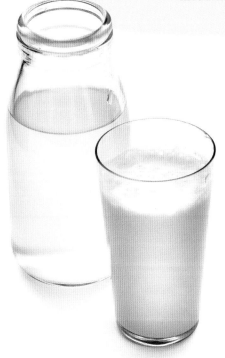

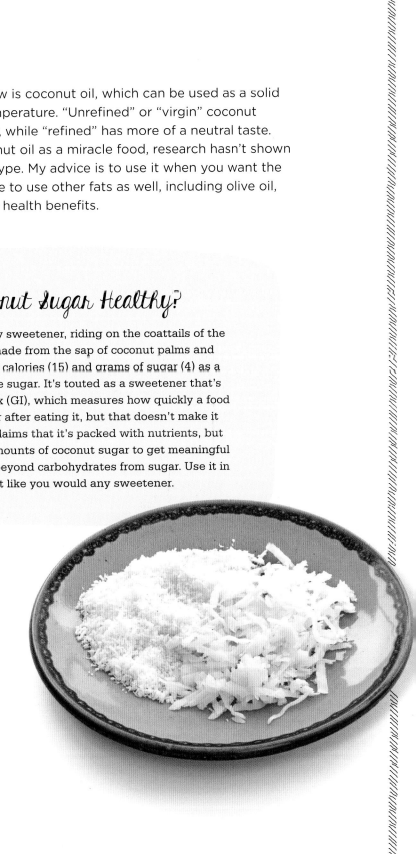

Dates

Dates may not be refreshing or loaded with vitamin C like other fruits. But what they do have is an intense sweetness that can satisfy a sweet tooth just as well as a candy bar. Dates are a great way to lend a natural sweetness to recipes, rather than adding sugar or a liquid sweetener such as honey or maple syrup. Two Medjool dates have thirty grams of (natural) sugar, the equivalent of about seven teaspoons.

Along with that natural sugar comes a handful of important nutrients. They are a **good source of potassium** and fiber and contain some iron and calcium. They're also **high in niacin**, a B vitamin that helps your child's body convert food into fuel. Dates also have **antioxidant powers**. In fact, in a study published in the *Journal of the American College of Nutrition* investigating the antioxidant potency of different foods, dates came out on top among all dried fruits.

Dates, which grow in clusters on palm trees, have been cultivated and enjoyed for thousands of years in the Middle East, and some varieties are now grown in the United States too (one of the most popular varieties is the Medjool). You can buy dates pitted or unpitted. Remove the pit by gently squeezing the date to push out the pit, or cut the date in half and remove. You can serve them plain or fill the space left by the pit with a walnut or dab of cream cheese. Since they are sticky and can cling to teeth, have your children brush after snacking on them (or swish with water). I keep dates on hand to blend into snack balls and smoothies. They're so intensely sweet that you won't need any added sweeteners such as honey or maple syrup.

My trick to fully pulverizing them in smoothies: Place a few dates in a small dish, cover with milk (dairy or nondairy), and allow them to soak in the refrigerator overnight. They'll be soft and easily blended in time for your morning drink.

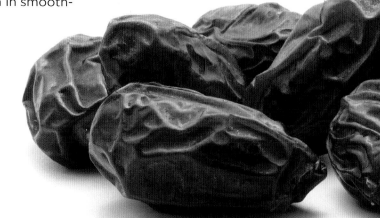

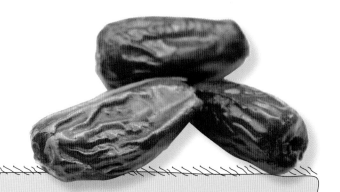

HELP!
My Kid Is Hooked on Sugar!

First, keep in mind that a preference for sweet foods is something everyone is born having, so it's natural. Some kids may be more sugar-crazy than others, but there are things you can do to cut back:

Go halfsies: Combine sweetened and unsweetened cereal, oatmeal, and even flavored and unflavored milk to keep some sweetness but reduce the overall added sugar.

Read labels: Sugar is in a lot of foods that don't even seem sweet. Start comparing products and switch to lower- or no-sugar versions of items such as crackers, salad dressings, and sauces.

Sweeten foods yourself: Even if you add a whole teaspoon (four grams) of sugar or honey to oatmeal or cereal, you'll still get much less than you would with most presweetened cereal and instant oatmeal.

Find a balance: Pay attention to the sugar your child gets each day. If she had cookies at preschool, skip dessert in favor of fruit after dinner. If you're going to a birthday party later, serve eggs instead of pancakes with syrup for breakfast that day.

Stick to water and milk: The top source of added sugar in a child's diet is sugary beverages such as soda, fruit punch, sweetened teas, and sports drinks. If you want to lower your child's intake of sugar, limiting those is the best place to start.

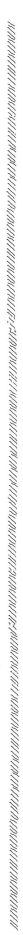

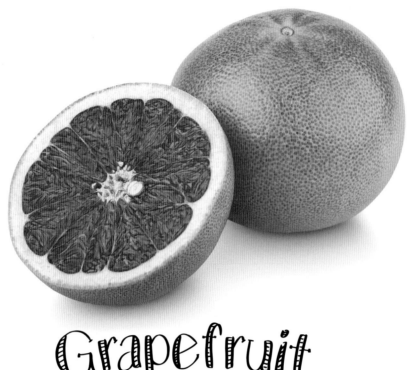

Grapefruit

If your kid's a fan of mouth-puckering gummies, tell him that grapefruit is nature's original sour candy. Maybe he'll roll his eyes—or maybe he'll try it and like it! Either way, it's worth a shot. And it's not the end of the world if you sprinkle half a grapefruit with a little bit of sugar or drizzle it with honey to sweeten the deal.

Grapefruit is **loaded with vitamin C**, which bolsters the immune system, keeps gums healthy, helps cuts and wounds heal properly, and acts as a free-radical–squashing antioxidant. Just one half of a medium grapefruit has all the C your child needs for the entire day. And if you're worried about your child getting enough iron, keep in mind that vitamin C helps the body better absorb this mineral. So eating C-rich and iron-rich foods together, such as having grapefruit and oatmeal at breakfast, will naturally help your child soak up more iron (grapefruit juice is packed with C but is missing the fiber of the whole fruit). Grapefruit also contains potassium and **lots of water to keep kids hydrated**. Pink and red varieties contain **beta-carotene and lycopene** as well, plant pigments that give them their color and have unique health-boosting properties.

When buying grapefruit, choose fruit that feels heavy—that means it will be juicy. They're picked when they're ripe, so they're ready right away. They'll keep in your refrigerator's crisper drawer for up to two weeks but taste sweeter if they're closer to room temperature. Rinse them before cutting so you don't drag any dirt from the outside into the flesh when slicing.

Broiled Grapefruit

A little bit of sugar can make sour grapefruit a little more enticing.

1 grapefruit
1 teaspoon brown sugar

Preheat the broiler to high. Cut the grapefruit in half (across the middle, not stem-end to stem-end) and remove any large seeds. Sprinkle each half evenly with the brown sugar. Place the halves on a baking sheet and broil for 3 to 5 minutes, or until the sugar bubbles. Serve warm.

Yield: 2 servings

Good to Know

Grapefruit can interfere with some medications. If your child regularly takes medicine, check with your doctor about whether there could be an interaction.

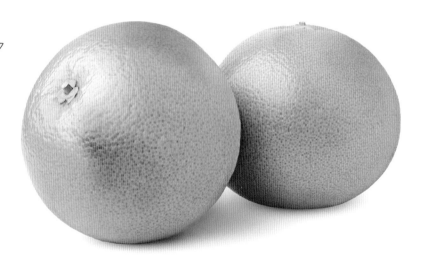

Grapes

Wine gets tons of hype for being healthy (handy justification for pouring a second glass!), but the truth is that fresh grapes are an incredible source of the same compounds—in a much kid-friendlier form.

Eaten for thousands of years, grapes make appearances in both the Bible and Egyptian hieroglyphics. Today the vast majority of "table grapes" (the kind we eat fresh) are grown in California, which produces more than eighty-five different varieties. No matter what color or kind of grape you buy, they all have health benefits because they contain polyphenols, natural plant compounds that help protect health. One of these polyphenols, called resveratrol, is found in high amounts in green, red, and black varieties of grapes and has been studied for **heart health benefits** and **anticancer powers**. Red and purple grapes get their color from another plant chemical called anthocyanins, pigments that act as antioxidants in the body. Grapes are **high in vitamin K**, which helps blood clot normally. And since they're more than 80 percent water, grapes are refreshing and hydrating.

Grapes are sold fully ripe and don't get any riper (or sweeter) once they're picked. When shopping, don't be turned off by a white, powdery covering on fresh grapes—it's not pesticide residue or dirt. It's called bloom, and it's the grapes' natural defense against moisture loss and decay. It tells you the grapes are fresh. Once you get your grapes home, remove any rotten grapes from the bunch and store the rest unwashed in a plastic bag in the refrigerator. They'll keep for up to two weeks that way. Or give them a rinse and place them on the counter for your kids to grab. (Just don't put them close to onions or leeks—the grapes will absorb their odors!)

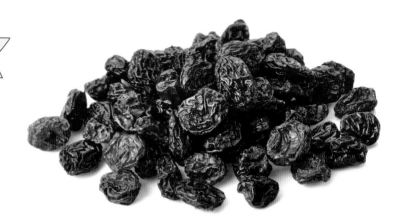

Good to Know

Whole grapes are considered a choking hazard for children younger than four. Slice grapes in half (large grapes may need to be quartered).

RAISINS

Raisins are a smart pick because unlike most dried fruit, they don't usually contain any added sugar. That's because raisins are naturally sweet (and fun fact: It's true that most of them are still dried by the sun!). A quarter-cup (35 g) serving of raisins is a **good source of iron for kids** and provides some fiber and potassium too. Research has even shown that raisins contain compounds that may help block the bacteria that cause cavities. (But it's still smart to swish with water or brush teeth after eating sticky foods.)

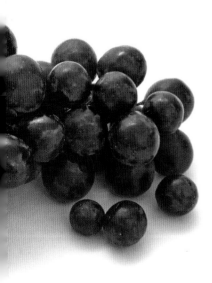

 "TRY IT" TIP

If your kids don't like the texture of fresh grapes, try freezing them—they taste like little bites of sorbet! Just remove them from the stem, rinse, and place on a baking sheet in a single layer in the freezer until firm. Then transfer them to a freezer bag or container to grab anytime.

Kiwifruit

Legend has it that this little fruit, native to China, was originally called a Chinese gooseberry. But a fruit dealer in the United States who was importing them from New Zealand began calling them kiwifruit, for the small brown New Zealand national bird, and the nickname stuck.

Fuzzy and brown on the outside and vibrant green on the inside, kiwi has a sweet-tart flavor. Each little kiwi has **more vitamin C than a kid needs in a whole day** and is a good source of potassium and fiber. Kiwi also contains an enzyme called actinidin, which may **help digestion by breaking down protein**. You'll get even more nutrients if you eat the skin too—yes, it's edible! (Just rinse it well first.)

Kiwi are grown in different parts of the world, so they're available year-round. Ripe kiwi will give a little when pressed, but unripe fruit will be hard and sour, so leave them on the counter for a few days until they're soft. Unlike other fruit that's more delicate, kiwi will keep well in the fridge for up to a month. To slice one into pieces, cut off the ends and slice it or remove the skin first with a vegetable peeler.

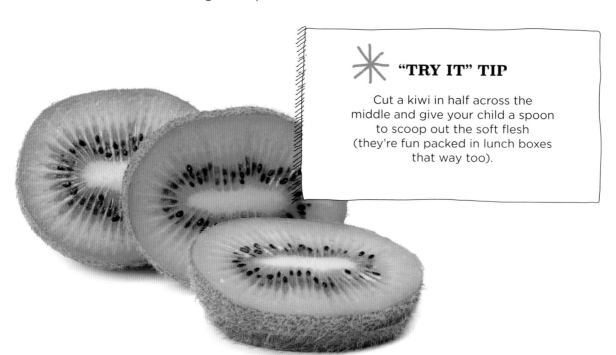

✳ "TRY IT" TIP

Cut a kiwi in half across the middle and give your child a spoon to scoop out the soft flesh (they're fun packed in lunch boxes that way too).

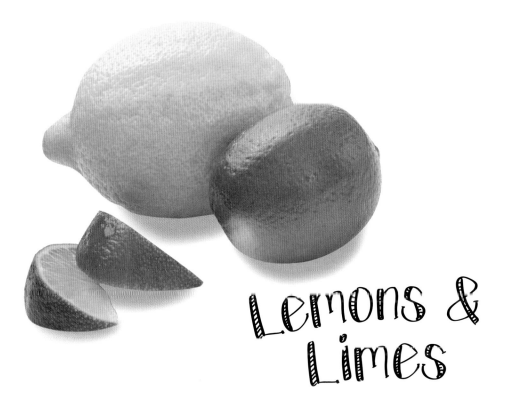

Lemons & Limes

Your child likely won't be eating slices of lemons and limes straight-up (except for my younger son, who has a strange habit of sucking on lemon wedges and making the rest of us cringe!). But keep the little citrus fruits around to add flavor to foods and drinks. They're a simple, sodium-free way to season recipes. Adding slices of lemons and limes to a pitcher of ice water adds flavor without sugar and may encourage kids to drink more.

Lemons and limes are both nutritious too. Both citrus fruits are **excellent sources of vitamin C**. There's also a protective compound in lemons called limonene that may have **anticancer powers** and plant chemicals called flavonol glycosides in limes that work as **antioxidants**, protecting cells from damage that can cause disease.

Good to Know

Meyer lemons are a cross between lemons and mandarin oranges. Compared to regular lemons, they're smaller, with darker-colored skin. They also have a much sweeter taste.

When buying lemons, look for ones that are bright, heavy, and medium to large in size. For lemons, opt for fruit with thin, smooth skin (very rough skin is a sign that there's more skin and less juice in each one). For limes, avoid fruit with blemishes or shriveled skin. You'll get more juice out of each lemon or lime if you bring them to room temperature before squeezing (or roll them on the counter to soften them). Got extra citrus juice after making a recipe? Freeze it in ice cube trays, then pop out and place in freezer bags for later.

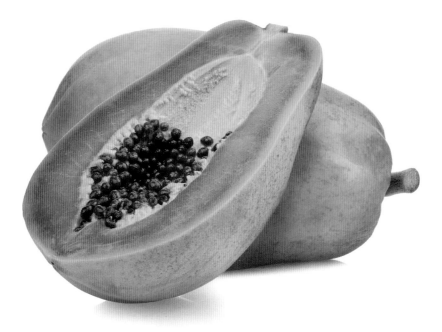

Papaya

Though the pineapple is probably one of the most familiar tropical fruits to kids, the papaya is so nutritious and tasty that it deserves some extra love too. Also called a pawpaw, papayas are a tropical fruit that hails from Mexico and Central America. Oblong like pears but much larger in size, papayas grow in clusters on tall plants that are actually herbs. The skin starts out green but turns yellow as it ripens. The flesh is a brilliant yellow-orange and tastes both sweet and tangy.

Papayas are **loaded with vitamins A and C**, important immune-boosting nutrients. They're also a **good source of folate**, potassium, and fiber. Like tomatoes, papayas contain lycopene, a pigment that gives the fruit its colors and is being studied for **cancer-fighting potential**. Plus, papayas contain cryptoxanthin, a carotenoid that's also associated with a reduced risk of some cancers.

When choosing one, look for yellow skin and fruit that gives slightly when pressed, or ripen it at home on the counter in a paper bag. When ready to eat, cut the papaya in half and scoop out the seeds (they are actually edible but bitter). Discard the skin and cut the flesh into slices or chunks for a fruit salad or to blend into a tropical smoothie. Or dice it up to add to fruit salsas. Papayas contain an enzyme called papain that naturally breaks down protein, so it's handy for meat marinades too.

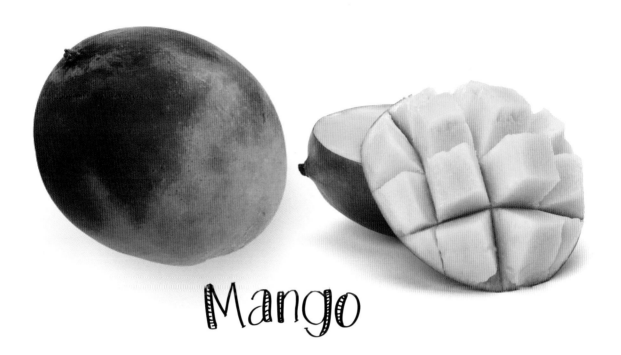

Mango

I didn't taste mango until I was in college, when I was on vacation in a tropical destination where we could pick the fruit straight from the trees. As I ate wedge after wedge, all I could think was, *I can't believe what I've been missing out on!*

A ripe mango is juicy and sweet-tart. It's **rich in vitamin C**, with a full day's supply for young kids. It's a good source of **immunity-boosting vitamin A** and the mineral potassium, which helps keep blood pressure at a healthy level. It also contains fiber for fullness and regularity and plenty of refreshing fluid for hydration. Thanks to its vibrant yellow flesh, it's also **rich in beta-carotene**, a pigment that works like an antioxidant to protect cells from damage.

A cousin to cashews and pistachios, mangoes grow on trees in tropical climates. Because there are several varieties with different growing seasons, you'll find them year-round in markets. When choosing one, keep in mind that color isn't a sign of ripeness. Instead, press gently. If the mango gives a bit, it's ripe (if not, keep it on the counter for a few more days). You can slice them up fresh to eat or dice them to add sweetness to fish tacos or fruit salsas you can serve with chicken and fish. Mango is a natural tenderizer, so it works well in marinades too. A bag of frozen mango chunks is also handy for giving morning smoothies a sweet, tropical twist.

Good to Know

If your child is sensitive or allergic to poison ivy or poison oak, don't let her handle mango skin. A chemical found in poison ivy and oak called urushiol is also found in mango skin and can cause rashes in sensitive people.

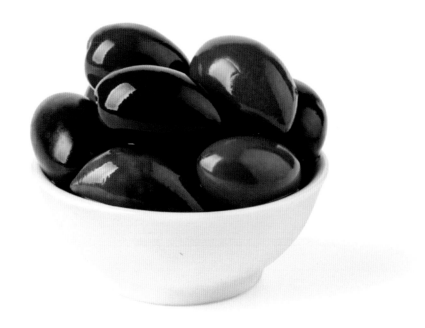

Olives

They may be more savory than sweet, but olives are technically a fruit. An ancient food that grows on a tree and contains a pit inside, olives are eaten whole or pressed to extract the oil in their flesh. And either way, they're a super-healthy food thanks to their abundance of **healthy fats**. Most of the fat in olives is monounsaturated, the kind that can help lower "bad" LDL cholesterol and **raise "good" HDL cholesterol**. Olives also contain several natural compounds that work as antioxidants, **protecting cells from disease-causing damage**.

Olives and olive oil are cornerstones of the Mediterranean Diet, a pattern of eating seen in countries bordering the Mediterranean Sea that's centered around fruits, vegetables, nuts, seeds, fish, seafood, whole grains, and healthy fats such as avocados and olive oil. After it was observed that people in these regions lived longer, healthier lives, the Mediterranean Diet has been widely studied. Researchers have found that this eating style has the potential to lower the risk for heart disease, certain kinds of cancer, and diabetes.

Should you go for black or green? They're actually the same kind of olive, just at different degrees of ripeness (green is less ripe). Olives are too bitter to be eaten straight off the tree, so they're cured in brine, salt, or olive oil. Black olives tend to taste milder than green. Add them to pizza and salads or let your kids stick them on the end of their fingers and pop them into their mouths one by one. Keep in mind that because olives are cured, they're high in sodium, so just keep an eye on other high-sodium foods your child is getting that day. Thankfully, just a few olives pack a big punch of flavor.

Q: Is Salt Bad for Kids?

Kids, like adults, are getting more sodium each day than the American Heart Association recommends. Because kids are facing problems formerly reserved for grown-ups such as high blood pressure, it's smart to keep an eye on intake. Most of the sodium both kids and adults get comes from processed, packaged, and restaurant foods. Only a small fraction stems from the saltshaker at home. So the best way to scale back is to buy fewer packaged snacks and high-sodium processed foods such as frozen dinners. But don't hold back on sprinkling a bit of kosher salt on roasted veggies or other dishes—it can bring out the flavor and make healthy foods even more appealing.

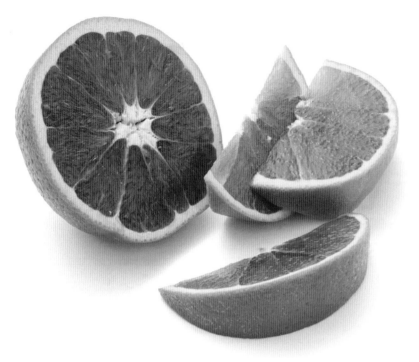
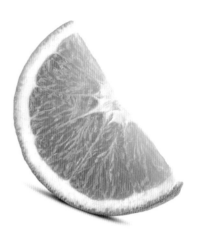

Oranges

Consider the orange **one-stop-shopping for vitamin C**. A medium orange has all the vitamin C an adult needs in a day—and at least double what kids need. It is also a **good source of folate** and contains potassium, which can **help keep blood pressure at healthy levels**, and each one offers three grams of fiber.

Navel oranges are the most popular oranges for eating, since they have no seeds and thick, easy-to-peel skin. Your store may also carry Valencia oranges, which have a thinner skin, and blood oranges, named for their red flesh. Blood oranges get their hue from anthocyanins, which work as antioxidants in the body. But hands-down the most kid-friendly kind of orange is the mandarin, a cinch for even young kids to peel by themselves (clementines are a seedless variety of mandarins).

Though I'm not a huge fan of juice for kids, 100 percent orange juice is definitely a better pick in my book than most because it's so high in potassium, folate, and vitamin C. Some varieties are also fortified with calcium and vitamin D, which some kids may be lacking (especially those who don't drink milk). Research shows that kids and adults who drink orange juice have higher intakes of vitamin C, calcium, and folate. But because it is also a concentrated source of natural sugar and lacks the fiber of whole oranges, stick to the guidelines set by the American Academy of Pediatrics (see page 71) by limiting your child's daily portion.

Juice that's labeled "not from concentrate" means that it was squeezed, (usually) pasteurized, and poured into containers. "From concentrate" means that some water was removed after squeezing, creating a concentrated form (like you'd get in a can of frozen juice concentrate in the freezer section), then water was added back in before packaging. There may be a difference in flavor between the two, but one isn't healthier than the other.

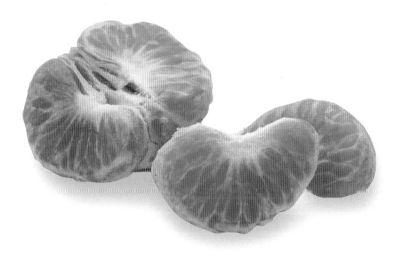

Better-for-You Orange Julius

Whip up this sweet, frothy drink that's a healthier take on the food court classic. While you're sipping, regale your kids with stories about the good ol' days when the mall was *the* place to be.

¾ cup (175 ml) milk
½ cup (115 g) vanilla yogurt
1 fresh orange, peeled
4 cubes frozen 100 percent orange juice (place orange juice in a standard ice cube tray—about 1 tablespoon [15 ml] per cube—and freeze until firm)
1 tablespoon (20 g) maple syrup

Place the milk, yogurt, orange, juice cubes, and maple syrup in a high-speed blender in the order listed. Blend under smooth, pour into 2 glasses, and serve immediately.

Yield: 2 servings

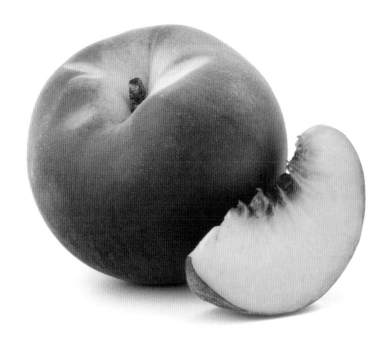

Peaches

Have you noticed that today's peaches aren't as fuzzy as they used to be? That's because growers are now "defuzzing" peaches mechanically to create a smoother skin. (Don't worry: It's not a scary, chemical-filled process, just a rubdown!) But if you're feeling nostalgic, you'll still find fuzzy peaches at the farmers' market. And if they're just-picked, they're also probably fresher and sweeter than what you might find in the supermarket.

Though they may not have the same lengthy résumé of health benefits as other fruits in this book, peaches are sweet and familiar to kids. They're also a **good source of vitamin C** and provide vitamin A, magnesium, and **potassium**. Each medium peach also supplies **two grams of fiber** for fullness and fighting constipation.

When buying peaches, avoid any that are rock-hard or have dark spots or green-tinted skin (a red flag they were picked too soon!). Look for peaches with skin that's yellow with shades of pink and red, and that smell fruity. Depending on the variety, the flesh may be either yellow or white, and they may have a pit that comes out easily (called freestone) or sticks to the flesh (called clingstone). To easily remove the pit in a freestone peach, use the same method as cutting an avocado: Slice all around the seed and twist the halves to open. Ripe peaches will give easily when pressed. Set them on the counter in a paper bag to speed the ripening process.

If you're buying canned peaches, choose ones packed in juice, not syrup, to avoid added sugar. When choosing frozen, look for bags that contain only peaches (and no added sugar). Peaches are perfect for eating out of hand like apples, slicing onto yogurt or oatmeal, or blending into smoothies. For a fun dessert, brush halved peaches with butter and grill them for a few minutes on each side. Serve with a scoop of ice cream or vanilla yogurt.

Q: Is it Okay for Kids to Snack?

Yes. Kids' smaller bellies and appetites mean they may need to eat more frequently to get the nourishment they need. But it's also easy for snacking to get out of control. Nonstop nibbling throughout the day means your child may not be hungry at mealtime—and that can be frustrating. If your children are munching on low-nutrient foods such as cheese-flavored crackers and granola bars, they may not be getting the vitamins and minerals (including iron and calcium) they need while they're growing. Ideally, it's best to schedule one or two snacks a day, well outside mealtimes, and serve a healthy, filling snack that will tide them over until the next meal. Some ideas: yogurt and fruit, hummus and carrots, or nut butter and whole grain crackers.

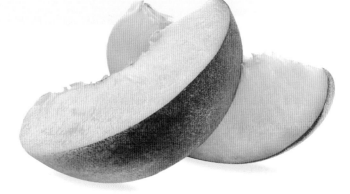

Pears

If there are any perks to summer coming to an end, pears are definitely one of them. Starting in late summer and early fall, pear varieties are in peak season and crop up on store shelves. Don't be discouraged if pears feel rock-hard at the market. They're sold unripe so they don't bruise or decay on shelves. After a day or two on the counter, they'll ripen and become soft, juicy, and sweet. How to know for sure: Press gently on the stem end of the pear with your thumbs. If it "gives," it's ready to eat. Want to speed the process? Put pears in a fruit bowl with bananas, which give off ethylene gas that speeds ripening. If your pears are ready but you're not, refrigerating them will slow the ripening.

Pears are **one of the highest fiber fruits**: There are six grams of fiber in one medium pear, a quarter of what kids need each day! Though pears contain some soluble fiber (the kind that may help lower cholesterol levels), they have more insoluble fiber—that's the kind that **helps prevent constipation**, which is a big problem for lots of kids. They're also a **good source of vitamin C**. Research published in the *Journal of Nutrition and Food Sciences* found that people who eat pears have higher intakes of fiber, vitamin C, magnesium, copper, and potassium (and lower intakes of added sugar) compared to people who don't eat them. Pears also contain a starch called pectin that works as a prebiotic in the gut, feeding the healthy bacteria that keep harmful bacteria at bay.

Good to Know

Like apples, sliced pears will brown when exposed to air, so slice them just before serving. If you need to chop them in advance, a squeeze of lemon juice (or dipping pieces into a mixture of water and lemon juice) will help slow the browning process.

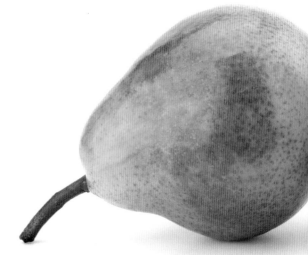

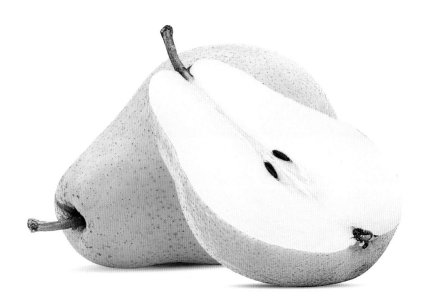

There are ten varieties of pears that grow in the United States, and they're all slightly different in taste, texture, and appearance—from Red Bartlett to Green Anjou. You can slice up fresh pears as a snack or chop them onto yogurt, oatmeal, and salads. Or halve them, scoop out the core, drizzle with a little honey, and bake them. However you serve them, try not to peel away the skin; it's where a lot of the nutrients are found. And if you're choosing canned pears, look for varieties canned in juice, not syrup, to avoid added sugar.

Good to Know

A teaspoon of sugar is the equivalent of four grams of sugar. Use this quick calculation when reading labels. For instance, a cereal with twelve grams of sugar per serving contains three teaspoons of sugar in each serving. But remember that dairy products and fruit both contain natural sugar—a kind that's not a concern for health—so even plain milk and unsweetened applesauce will list some sugar on the label.

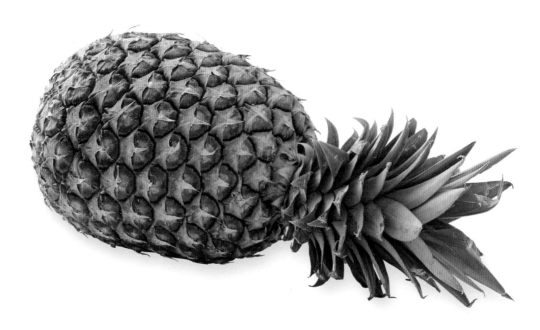

Pineapple

True story: After hearing that eating pineapple before surgery helps reduce swelling, I ate it every day for a week before having two wisdom teeth pulled at the dentist's office. The result? Absolutely no telltale "chipmunk cheeks." I can't say for sure that it was the pineapple, but the tropical fruit is a food source of bromelain, an enzyme that is thought to have **anti inflammatory powers**. (Bromelain also breaks down protein, so it's perfect for a quick, tenderizing meat marinade too!)

Pineapple comes from a Spanish word meaning "pinecone" because of its prickly exterior. It's a good source of fiber and an **excellent source of vitamin C**. One cup of chunks has as much vitamin C as a medium orange. It's also **rich in manganese**, a mineral that helps the body get energy from food.

Pineapples are picked ripe, so you can eat them right after purchasing. When choosing a fresh one, look for green leaves (not brown) and avoid any with bruises or bad spots. It should smell sweet and fruity if it's at room temperature. Keep whole pineapples in the refrigerator until you're ready to cut them. When buying canned pineapple, get a variety packed in juice (not syrup) to avoid added sugar. I like to use the leftover juice to sweeten smoothies or make ice pops: If you don't have reusable molds, pour the juice into paper cups, cover with plastic wrap, then insert a popsicle stick through the wrap and into the juice. When the pop is frozen, remove the plastic wrap and peel away the cup.

HOW TO CUT A WHOLE PINEAPPLE

There are several schools of thought on this, but here's how I do it: Trim off the stem end and the bottom. Stand the pineapple upright and slice down along the sides, cutting away the rind. Trim off any remaining "eyes" on the pineapple's flesh. Now make four vertical cuts top to bottom around the center core. Discard the core and chop the quarters into slices or cubes.

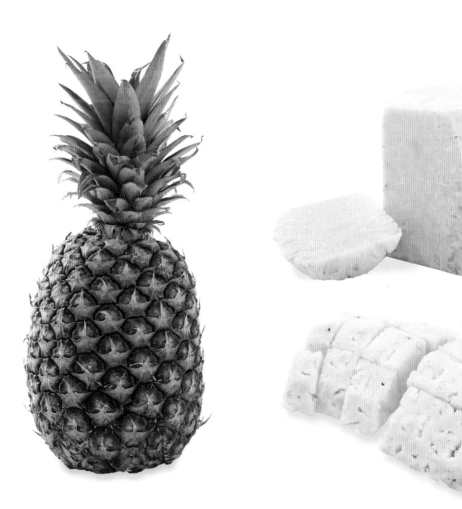

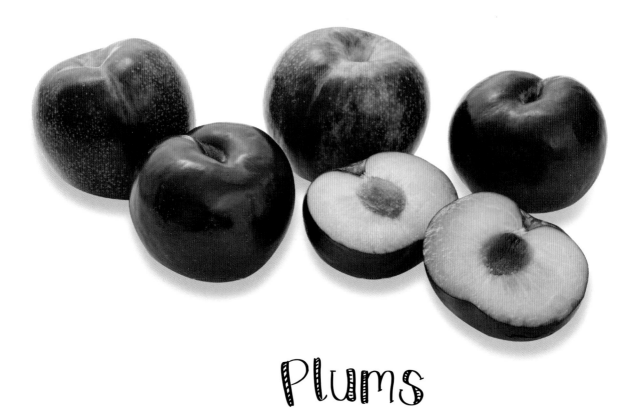

Plums

Sweet, juicy plums come in hundreds of varieties, and more than one hundred of them are available in the United States, typically during the summer months. Plums are drupes, which means they have a pit inside like peaches and apricots. Some plums are freestone, meaning the pit can easily be removed, while others are clingstone, with flesh that clings to the pit. The skin of plums ranges from blue and green to red and almost black, and the flesh inside can be red, green, or yellowish. Plums are a **good source of vitamin C**, with a **high water content** that makes them refreshing.

When choosing plums, select fruit that's either firm or that yields a bit to pressure. Avoid any with shriveled skin or that feel mushy. Keep them on the counter to ripen. If you're antsy, place them in a paper bag to speed ripening. You can keep them refrigerated once they're ripe, but they'll taste sweeter if they're closer to room temperature. Around here, we bite right into plump, round plums like apples. You can also slice them up and eat them as a snack or chop them over yogurt or salads.

PRUNES

Prunes are simply dried plums, and they're usually processed without any added sugar or sulfates. Prunes' claim to fame is relieving constipation, and that's likely due to two things: Half the fiber they contain is insoluble, the kind that pulls water into the intestines to make stools softer and easier to pass. Plus, they contain sorbitol, a sugar alcohol that also soaks up water in the digestive tract. In fact, research has found that prunes are just as **effective at fighting constipation** as store-bought fiber supplements. Like raisins, prunes are also a **good source of iron**. You can pulse prunes in the food processor (along with some hot water) and make a prune purée to use in recipes in place of some of the butter or oil, as you would applesauce. And FYI for shoppers: Prunes have recently been rebranded by some companies, so you may see the term "dried plums" on packages instead.

 "TRY IT" TIP

If your kids balk at the idea of trying prunes, look for diced dried plums. They look more like raisins than prunes, so they seem familiar. They can be eaten right out of hand or tossed into trail mixes and onto cereal.

Pomegranate

This fruit may have been eaten for thousands of years—it was a favorite among Egyptian pharaohs, and a pomegranate-shaped vase was found in King Tut's tomb!—but it's still a mystery to a lot of people today. Called the Jewel of the Winter, the pomegranate looks like it's wearing a crown, and inside that hard, leathery exterior are plump, juicy seeds that are worth the effort it takes to get them out.

Whole pomegranates have a limited growing season (typically October to January in the United States), so stock up while you can. The fruit will actually last for months tucked into the fridge or about a month on the counter. You don't eat the hard exterior—getting to the bright red seeds inside, called arils, is the goal here. Juicy and tart-sweet, the arils are a **great source of fiber and vitamin C** for kids and are fun to eat right out of hand or to sprinkle on top of yogurt or oatmeal. They also contain antioxidants called polyphenols that **protect the cells from free radical damage**. When shopping, look for pomegranates that feel heavy for their size, and don't stress about finding the reddest one, since color is no reflection of how sweet and tasty the seeds will be.

Pomegranate juice, sold year-round, packs **as much potassium per serving as a banana**, and researchers are studying possible links between the juice and improved memory and better recovery after exercise in adults. The juice is made by pressing the entire fruit, so you'll nab the antioxidants in the seeds, rind, and pulp that way. Add some juice to a smoothie or a splash to a glass of seltzer to make an easy, low-sugar spritzer (but as with all juices, stick to the American Academy of Pediatrics guidelines, discussed on page 71).

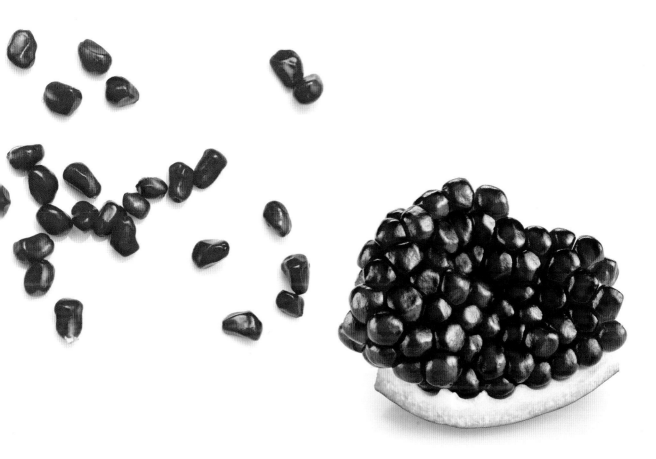

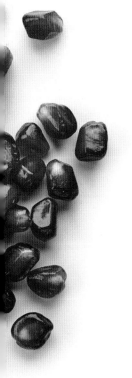

HOW TO SEED A POMEGRANATE

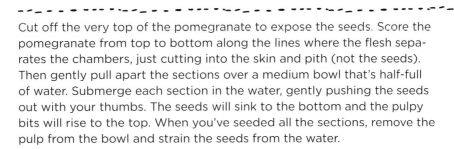

Cut off the very top of the pomegranate to expose the seeds. Score the pomegranate from top to bottom along the lines where the flesh separates the chambers, just cutting into the skin and pith (not the seeds). Then gently pull apart the sections over a medium bowl that's half-full of water. Submerge each section in the water, gently pushing the seeds out with your thumbs. The seeds will sink to the bottom and the pulpy bits will rise to the top. When you've seeded all the sections, remove the pulp from the bowl and strain the seeds from the water.

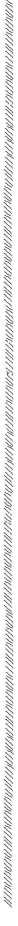

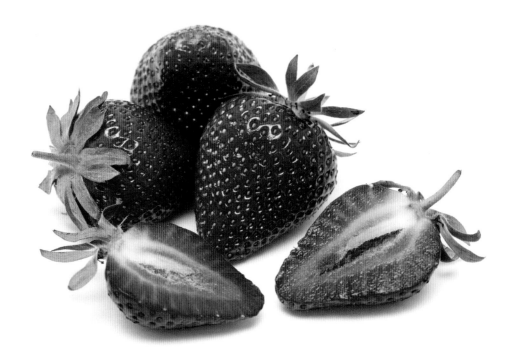

Strawberries

A young child can get her entire day's worth of vitamin C by eating just *three* medium berries (so don't be fooled by sugary drinks and snacks with labels that boast "100% vitamin C!" as if it's hard to come by in actual, real food!). In fact, strawberries actually pack more C than oranges, ounce for ounce. Vitamin C is known as an **immune system superhero** because it boosts the body's production of antibodies to squash foreign invaders. Strawberries **rank among the top ten fruits in antioxidant capacity**, which measures the ability of the food's components to destroy free radicals. Because it's a water-soluble vitamin, C doesn't get stored in the body (any extra literally gets flushed out in the bathroom), so it's a nutrient kids need to get every day.

With three grams of filling fiber per half cup (73 g), strawberries are a rich source of folate, a B vitamin that helps protect heart health. Strawberries also contain natural plant compounds that may work together to fight cancer. In research published in the *Journal of Agriculture and Food Chemistry,* the berries' phenolic compounds were shown to inhibit the growth of oral, prostate, and colon cancer cells. Certain tannins in strawberries have also been studied in animals and lab tests for their **anticancer powers**, and researchers say the berries may help reduce the risk of developing diabetes and fight the kind of inflammation related to disease.

Be sure to wash your berries just before eating and store them in a single layer when possible.

➡ Melted Berry Sauce

Spoon a tablespoon of this sweet-tart sauce over your child's plain yogurt or oatmeal instead of buying presweetened kinds. You'll get plenty of sweetness with all the nutrition of whole fruit.

⅓ cup (about 80 g) each frozen blueberries, strawberries,
**   and raspberries (or 1 cup [240 g] total of frozen berries of your choice)**
1 tablespoon (20 g) maple syrup

Combine the fruit in a small saucepan over medium-high heat, stirring as the fruit defrosts. Press the fruit with the back of your spoon to release the juices. Reduce the heat to medium-low, add the maple syrup, and continue cooking for 7 to 10 minutes, or until the mixture thickens, stirring constantly. Transfer the sauce to a glass jar or container and use warm or cold. If you prefer a smooth texture, purée the sauce in a blender or food processor.

Yield: About ½ cup (120 ml)

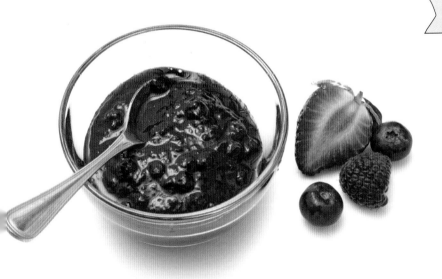

Good to Know

Some whole fruit actually does fine on the counter, such as apples, oranges, tomatoes, bananas, pineapple, and grapefruit. But keep in mind that bananas, apples, avocados, peaches, pears, and plums all produce a gas called ethylene. Pile them with other fruits in a bowl, and they'll speed ripening.

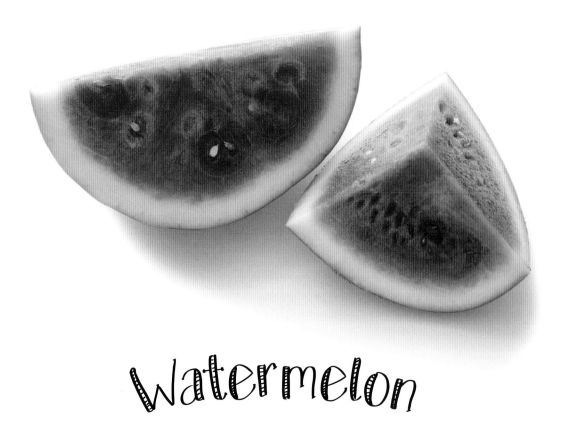

Watermelon

Is there any surer sign of summer than a kid with a slice of bright red watermelon, juice dripping down her arm? The timing of watermelon season couldn't be better: The fruit is 92 percent water, so it's **refreshing and hydrating** for steamy summer days. And though watermelon may not earn a spot in the Superfoods Hall of Fame, its nutritional stats aren't too shabby: One serving (a whopping two cups, or 300 grams, of diced melon) has **all the vitamin C young kids need in a day** and is a **good source of vitamin A**. The pigment that gives watermelon its color is called lycopene, an antioxidant that researchers are studying for its potential to inhibit cancer and even **protect the skin from UV rays**. There's also a little bit of fiber in each juicy bite.

Look for a melon that is heavy for its size (that means it's juicy) and has a creamy yellow or white spot (that means it's ripe). Ever bring home a melon only to discover that it's soft and mushy? If you can't return it to the market, purée the fruit into watermelon juice along with a squeeze of fresh lemon or lime juice. Or cut the melon into chunks and freeze. Once they're solid, pop them into the blender with a little bit of water or juice for an easy watermelon "sorbet." Fun fact: The watermelon rind is edible too! After eating a slice, cut the light green rind away from the peel and toss chunks of it into a blender or juicer along with the red watermelon flesh and a squeeze of honey.

HOW TO CUT WATERMELON "STICKS"

This is a fun, grab-and-go way to slice watermelon and works especially well for serving kids. Cut the watermelon across the middle (not stem to stem). Lay each half on a cutting board, cut-side down. Slice through the watermelon and cut into strips about two inches (5 cm) wide, then rotate the whole thing and cut into two-inch (5 cm) strips the other way. Pull out the "sticks" and serve.

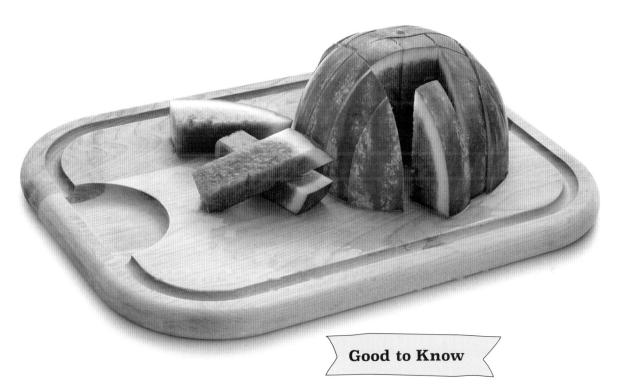

Good to Know

Though you may have memories of spitting watermelon seeds across the backyard, seedless varieties have become much more popular and widespread. Seedless melons are produced through hybridization (when two varieties are crossed), not genetic modification. Any white seeds you spot in a seedless watermelon are actually seed coatings and are totally edible.

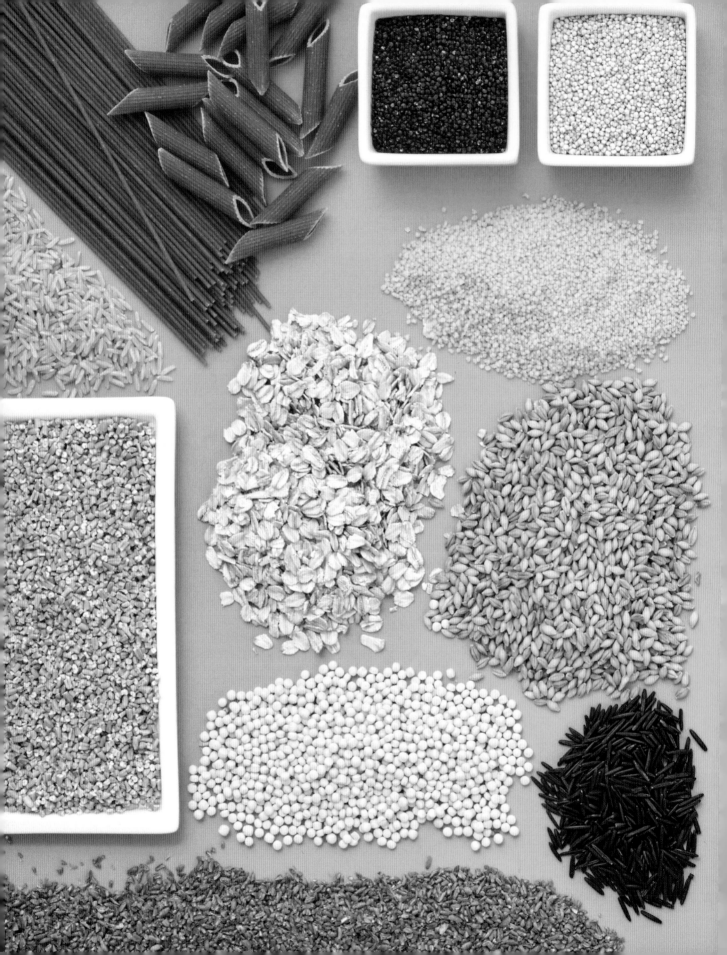

3

Grains

BE WARY OF ANY HEALTH GURU WHO SUGGESTS nixing grains from your child's diet. Grains are a rich source of carbohydrates, the body's main source of fuel, and kids need plenty of those to keep their bodies and brains going all day. Plus, there's a large body of research showing that whole grains (the kinds that haven't been stripped down and refined) are linked to a healthier body weight, better cholesterol levels, and reduced risk for heart disease. Whole grains also pack more fiber, minerals, and vitamins than the refined grains do—plus 25 percent more protein.

Ideally, at least half of your child's grains for the day should be whole. It's smart to get kids familiar with the taste, texture, and flavor of whole grains so they'll like them (and continue eating them throughout their lives!). But I get it: Not every kid is a fan of all of them right out of the gate, so balance it out. If your child had her PB&J on white for lunch, serve her whole grain crackers with cheese at snack time. If you have white pasta for dinner, offer brown rice tomorrow.

HOW MANY GRAINS DO YOUR KIDS NEED EVERY DAY?

- Ages 2–3: 3 ounces (85 g)
- Ages 4–8: 5 ounces (142 g)
- Ages 9–13: 5 ounces (142 g) (girls), 6 ounces (170 g) (boys)
- Ages 14–18: 6 ounces (170 g) (girls), 8 ounces (227 g) (boys)

   *1 ounce (28 g) = 1 slice bread, 1 cup (weight varies) cereal, or 1/2 cup (83 g) cooked rice or pasta

   *Weight varies. Source: United States Department of Agriculture (USDA)

Barley

Barley is the **highest fiber whole grain around**. Unfortunately, the most common form of barley that's eaten is pearled barley, which has been stripped of its bran coating, polished, and enriched with some of the vitamins and minerals lost during processing. Cream-colored and often found in soups, pearled barley is not considered a whole grain. But according to the Whole Grains Council, it's still much healthier than other refined grains because the fiber is distributed throughout the kernel (not just in the bran that's removed). In fact, it has a pretty respectable amount of fiber for a refined grain: three grams in just a half cup (77 g) of cooked barley. Barley also contains a kind of fiber called beta-glucan that not only **helps lower cholesterol levels** but may also help **strengthen the immune system** and reduce the risk for developing diabetes.

For true whole grain barley, check a natural food or health food store and look for the words "whole grain barley" on the package. Whole grain barley has the inedible hull removed but the bran intact, making it higher in fiber and richer in nutrients such as B vitamins and iron. It takes longer to cook than pearled barley, is chewier, and has a heartier flavor. You can add barley, whole grain or pearled, to soups such as beef barley (or mushroom barley if you're going meatless), pilaf, and cold grain salads.

Along with wheat and rye, barley contains gluten, a protein that some people can't tolerate. For people diagnosed with celiac disease, eating gluten causes the body's immune system to mount a defense and damage the intestines, making it harder to absorb nutrients from food. If your child has celiac disease or gluten intolerance, you'll want to avoid barley and any foods that contain it, including malt vinegar and malted beverages.

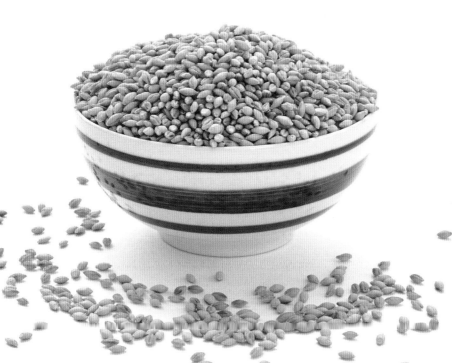

HELP!
My Kid Is Always Hungry!

When it comes to your children, does it seem like the requests for food never end? Appetites can surge during growth spurts (which is totally normal), but if it feels like you're *always* in the kitchen prepping food for your kids, ask yourself these questions.

Are your child's meals and snacks filling enough? Kids tend to gravitate toward foods such as pretzels and granola bars that aren't very satisfying. Try to include filling nutrients such as protein, healthy fats, and fiber in meals and snacks for more staying power.

Is your child just bored? Like adults, kids can eat out of boredom. Talk to your child about hunger and fullness and help her figure out how she really feels.

Is your child simply thirsty? Thirst can be mistaken for hunger, so be sure your child is drinking plenty of water throughout the day.

Brown Rice

White rice is a staple for populations around the world, but brown rice is the winner nutritionally. Unlike white rice, which has been stripped of its bran and germ layers, brown rice is the whole grain of rice (ditto for black, purple, and red rice). The only part that's missing is the outer, inedible husk. This means it has **double the fiber of white rice** and naturally higher amounts of vitamins and minerals. A kid-sized portion of cooked brown rice (one-half cup, or 100 grams) has about **two grams of fiber** and is a **good source of phosphorus**, magnesium, and **iron**.

Because it hasn't been stripped and refined, brown rice also has a heartier flavor and a chewier texture compared to white. Instant brown rice tends to be a bit less chewy than regular brown rice, so that's a good place to start with white rice diehards. My kids like brown rice as a bed for stir-fries. Or you can serve build-your-own Buddha bowls: Give everyone a bowl of cooked brown rice and let them serve themselves from bowls of toppings such as roasted veggies, baked tofu, leafy greens, and chopped nuts. Top it all with a drizzle of Easy Peanut Sauce (see page 183).

And rest assured that if your family likes only white rice (for now at least!), it still contains nutrients. Like many refined grains, white rice is enriched. That means that some of the nutrients that are lost during processing are added back in by fortification. So it's a good source of nutrients including iron and B vitamins. In an analysis published in *Nutrition Today*, children who ate rice (whether brown or white) took in more protein, vitamin A, B vitamins, iron, magnesium, copper, and potassium and less total and saturated fat than those who didn't eat rice.

Q: I've Heard There's Arsenic in Rice. Should I Be Worried?

Arsenic is a toxic element found in the soil, air, and water. The FDA, which tests arsenic levels in food, has concluded that rice tends to contain more arsenic than other foods because of the way the crop is grown. Since there's arsenic throughout the environment, you can't avoid it completely. But you can help minimize your exposure by serving a variety of grains and not relying on a single kind. The FDA also says that cooking rice in an excess of water and draining it (similar to how you cook pasta) can reduce up to 60 percent of the arsenic content.

Good to Know

"Parboiled" or "converted" rice means that the rice has been steamed before processing. That helps lock in some of the nutrients. "Instant" rice has been cooked and dehydrated, so it's speedy to prepare.

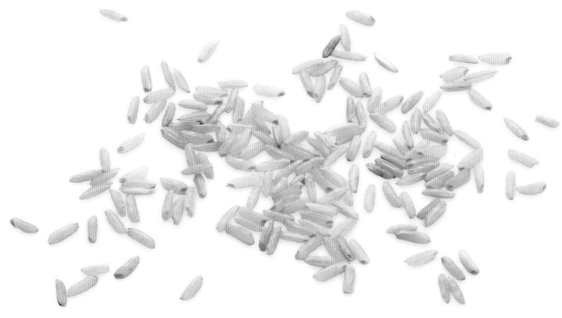

Bulgur

Whole grains such as bulgur are so helpful in your child's day because they deliver more fiber, protein, vitamins, and minerals than refined grains do. In just one-half cup (91 g) of cooked bulgur, your child will get **four grams of fiber** (young kids need about twenty grams of fiber for the whole day), **three grams of protein**, a **decent amount of iron**, plus zinc, magnesium, and phosphorus. And it's a nice change of pace from rice and other more mainstream grains.

Bulgur is created when kernels of wheat are cooked, dried, and cracked into small pieces. Since it's precooked, it's quick to prepare. You can either cook it in boiling water or broth as you would pasta, or you can simply pour boiling liquid over it (one part bulgur to two parts water), cover it, let it soak up the water and reconstitute, and drain off any excess liquid after about twenty minutes. Bulgur labeled "fine grain" will take less time to cook than "coarse grain."

The chewy, nutty-tasting grain is the star of tabbouleh, a Mediterranean cold salad made with chopped tomato and cucumber, lots of parsley, and a dressing of lemon or lime juice and olive oil. I like adding bulgur to lentil soup, and you can also include cooked bulgur in recipes for chili, stuffed peppers, muffins, and breads.

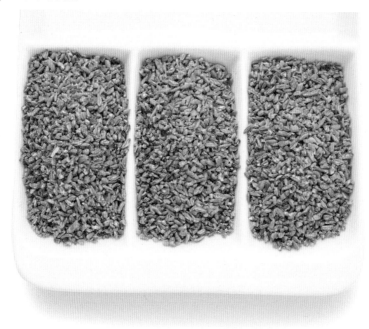

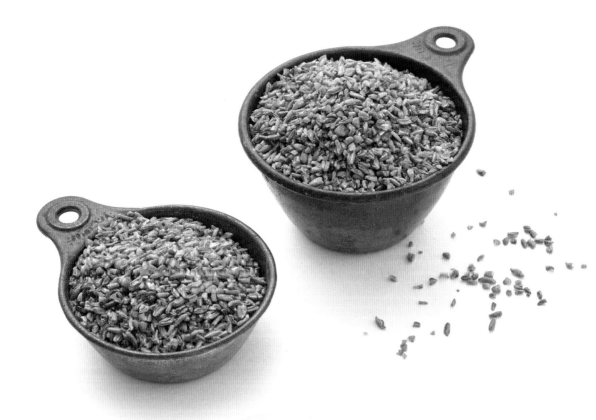

Read the fine print when "made with whole grain" is advertised on the package. In some cases, most of the grains are actually refined, and a whole grain may not appear until the third or fourth ingredient. If you want a truly whole grain product, look for the word "whole" (such as whole wheat) as the first ingredient.

Q: Is the Paleo Diet Safe for Kids?

Maybe—with many cautions. The Paleo Diet, based on the idea that we should eat only foods that our prehistoric ancestors could hunt and gather, centers around meat, fish, eggs, vegetables, and fruit but doesn't allow grains, beans, dairy, sugar, and highly processed packaged stuff. If it's very well planned, the diet might be able to supply the nutrients your kids need. But with no dairy, it's easy to skimp on calcium and vitamin D. With no grains, kids may not get the carbohydrates they need. And because it's heavy on meat and veggies, children could fill up before they've gotten enough calories. Since the diet is so restrictive, kids may also feel deprived and resentful if they're not allowed to eat the food at parties or friends' houses—and could end up sneaking or obsessing about food.

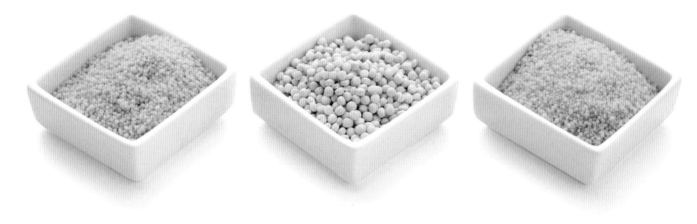

Couscous

Couscous is actually not a kind of grain itself but rather a type of pasta made from flour and water. Though most versions of it are made from refined white flour, you'll want to seek out "whole wheat" couscous to get more nutrition. A half cup (79 g) of cooked whole wheat couscous has **three grams of fiber** and a whopping **six grams of protein** and is a **good source of iron**. Since it's made from flour, it's not gluten free (so not an option if your child has celiac disease or is gluten intolerant).

Couscous, which hails from North Africa and is popular in Middle Eastern cuisine, has already been steamed and dried. That means it's a cinch to prep: Just boil a small pot of water, turn off the heat, add the dry couscous, and cover. It will absorb the water and be ready to serve in just a handful of minutes. It's lighter and fluffier than rice but can be used in the same way. Add it to soups and stews, or serve it with some butter or olive oil and seasonings as a side. I like serving it under chicken or fish with a pan sauce because it soaks up all the extra liquid.

You may also spot pearl couscous (sometimes called Israeli couscous). The pieces are larger and rounder than regular couscous, and instead of simply soaking it, you simmer it on the stove like rice. You can find pearl couscous in a whole wheat version too.

Q: Should We Avoid Gluten?

Not unless it's medically necessary for your child. Gluten is a protein found in wheat, barley, and rye. Children with celiac disease—an autoimmune disorder in which the body can't digest gluten—must avoid all gluten or suffer intestinal damage. Other kids may be diagnosed with non-celiac gluten sensitivity, which means they have symptoms such as bloating or headaches that get better when gluten is removed from their diets. Otherwise, it's not a nutritional villain, and cutting it out doesn't make their diets healthier. Gluten-free breads and snacks may pack more starch, fat, and sugar (and less fiber) than gluten-containing ones do. They're also typically more expensive. A gluten-free diet can be very challenging for kids too, since they can't have a lot of typical foods. Finally, keep in mind there's no evidence that delaying the introduction of gluten for babies helps prevent celiac disease.

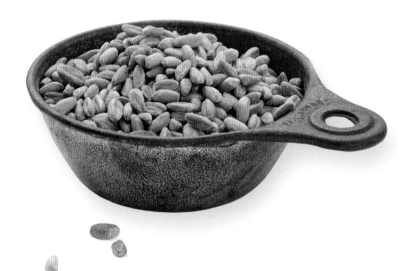

Farro

Farro is what's known as an ancient grain, which are grains that have been eaten for hundreds (if not thousands) of years and have remained relatively unchanged in that time. Ancient grains also usually haven't been refined, so they haven't been stripped or processed in a way that removes some of their nutrition. Farro, a whole grain and a kind of wheat, looks a lot like barley and has a nutty taste and a chewy texture.

Farro has **five grams of fiber** per three-quarter cup (90 g) cooked serving (that's about a quarter of what kids need in a day!) plus seven grams of protein. The fiber-protein combo makes farro an especially filling and satisfying grain. It's also an **excellent source of iron**, a mineral kids especially need while they're growing, and a little bit of calcium. Researchers have also found that farro is a **rich source of polyphenols**, plant chemicals that can protect against the kind of cell damage that leads to chronic diseases such as heart disease and cancer. Because it's a type of wheat, farro is not gluten free.

To prep farro, simmer it on the stove like rice. If you soak it in water for several hours or overnight first, you can cut the cooking time by two-thirds. Do your kids already like risotto? If so, make it using farro in place of Arborio rice next time. You can also add farro to soups and stews or bake it into casseroles.

Good to Know

Ancient grains are hot right now, and though they're typically nutritious, be wary of processed foods including breakfast cereals, bars, or chips that advertise "made with ancient grains." That doesn't necessarily mean they are healthy picks. You should still check the package for a relatively short, simple ingredient list. Be sure to check the sugar content too.

Millet

Yes, millet looks like bird food. And there's a very good reason for that: It actually *is* bird food. A common component of birdseed mixes sold in the United States, millet is an ancient grain that's been eaten (by people!) for thousands of years. Though it's a common food in many parts of the world, it's still unfamiliar to plenty of folks—but it deserves a place on your child's plate.

A whole grain, millet is a small, round, yellow grain that has a mild flavor and is naturally gluten free. A half-cup (87 g) serving of cooked millet has **three grams of filling fiber** and five grams of satisfying protein and is a **good source of iron and zinc**. Millet also contains magnesium, which can help regulate blood pressure, and phosphorus for strong teeth and bones. The grain has also been shown in research to have **high antioxidant activity**, which means it can help neutralize free radicals that travel through the body and damage cells. It's that kind of cellular damage that's thought to contribute to disease.

So what do you do with it? You can add millet straight out of the bag into homemade granola or muffin recipes. You can also simmer millet on the stove as you would with rice and serve it as a breakfast porridge, make it into a pilaf, or add it to soups and stews.

Q: How Much Fiber Does My Child Need?

In general, toddlers and preschoolers should have about twenty grams of fiber per day, older kids twenty-five grams. As with adults, most kids are falling woefully short—and getting enough is important. Fiber helps kids' systems run smoothly, warding off constipation. It keeps them full, so they're satisfied with meals and snacks. And fiber-rich foods such as whole grains and produce are packed with vitamins and minerals kids need for growth.

Just remember that if your child doesn't currently eat a lot of high-fiber foods, you should add them in slowly. A bunch of extra fiber at one time can cause gas and bloating.

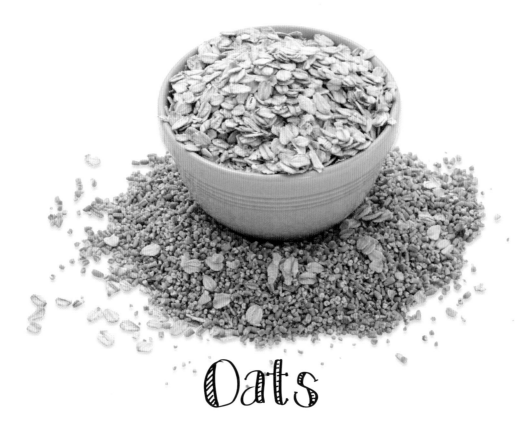

Oats

Oats are actually a **natural whole grain**. They don't get stripped of their bran or germ, so you can feel good that your kids are getting a whole grain, no matter what kind you buy. A quick primer: Rolled oats are steamed and flattened. Quick and instant oats are simply rolled oats that are cut into smaller pieces, so they cook faster. Steel-cut oats haven't been rolled at all, so they are chewier and take longer to cook (about 20 to 30 minutes on the stovetop). But all three of these oat types are 100 percent whole grain and have the same health benefits.

Oats are **rich in two kinds of fiber**: Insoluble fiber is the type that adds bulk to stools, making them easier to pass—so if your kids struggle with constipation (and a lot of kids do!), oats are a natural way to help relieve it. They also pack a soluble fiber called beta-glucan that **helps lower "bad" LDL cholesterol levels** by actually pulling some LDL out with it when it passes out of the body. Soluble fiber is also filling and slows digestion, which is why oats are a stick-with-you a.m. meal that can keep your kids full all morning.

Good to Know

Oats are naturally gluten free, but some are processed in the same facility as gluten-containing foods. So if you're avoiding gluten, look for oats specifically labeled "gluten free."

Make-Ahead Instant Oatmeal Packets

No doubt oatmeal packets are convenient—but they're typically loaded with added sugar and sometimes ingredients such as fake food dyes. You can easily make your own with whole food ingredients and customize them just the way your family likes them.

3 cups (240 g) quick oats
6 sandwich-sized resealable plastic bags
Variety of add-ins such as brown sugar, cinnamon,
  dried and freeze dried fruit, nuts, and seeds

Place 1 cup (80 g) of the oats in a blender or food processor and blend or process until a powder is formed. Place in a medium bowl along with the remaining 2 cups (160 g) of oats and stir to combine. Portion ½ cup (40 g) of the oats mixture into each of the bags and add a variety of mix-ins. To cook, pour the contents of a bag into a deep cereal bowl, add ½ cup (120 ml) milk, cover the bowl with a small plate, and microwave on high power for 1 to 1½ minutes. Stir in 1 to 2 teaspoons of honey or maple syrup if desired. Mix together and enjoy.

SOME FLAVOR IDEAS:
2 teaspoons brown sugar + ¼ teaspoon ground cinnamon
1 tablespoon (4 g) peanut powder + 2 teaspoons unsweetened cocoa powder
¼ cup (5 g) freeze-dried strawberries + 1 tablespoon (8 g) chopped walnuts
¼ cup (33 g) chopped dried apricots + 2 teaspoons chia seeds

Yield: 6 servings

Q: Are Carbs Unhealthy?

Carbohydrates have gotten a bad reputation in certain circles, and some dieters try to cut back on them as much as possible. It's true that a lot of junk foods and sweets are high in carbs. But carbohydrates are also found in highly nutritious foods including fruits, veggies, dairy products, beans, nuts, and whole grains. Carbohydrates are the main source of fuel for the body and brain, so don't restrict them for your kids.

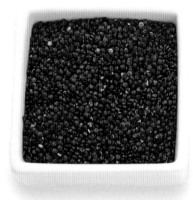 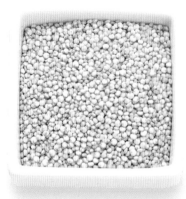 

Quinoa

Remember when nobody had heard of quinoa—or even knew how to pronounce it? (FYI, it's said like this: KEEN-wah.) It may seem like it was overnight success for quinoa, but quinoa is actually an ancient food that's been eaten for thousands of years (it was considered sacred to the Incas). Today the quinoa we eat is grown in the Andes Mountains of South America, and though it's often classified as a grain, it's technically a seed.

One reason for quinoa's popularity: **It's a complete protein**, containing all essential amino acids. That's rare for plant foods (most fall short on some of them) and good news for kids eating a vegetarian or vegan diet, because they can nab four grams of complete protein in each half-cup (93 g) of cooked quinoa. It's a **good source of fiber** and **gluten free** too, so children with celiac disease or gluten intolerance can safely eat it or products (such as pasta) made from it.

Though white is the most common color of quinoa you'll see in supermarkets, you may also spot red and black varieties. It cooks up in much the same way as rice does: You can cook it in water or (for more flavor) broth, and it's ready in about 15 minutes (be sure you rinse it before cooking to remove a natural coating that can taste bitter). The flavor is mild and sort of nutty, and you can serve it as a grain side dish, as you would rice or couscous, in cold salads, as a warm breakfast cereal, or baked into dishes such as casseroles and even bars and cookies.

Baked Quinoa Bites

These cheesy bites are a fun way to serve quinoa to your kids. If they don't dig broccoli, use a half cup of another veggie they like such as sweet red pepper or spinach. Or leave out veggies entirely at first and try again later.

Nonstick cooking spray, for preparing the muffin tin
2 cups (370 g) cooked and cooled quinoa (²/₃ cup [115 g] uncooked)
2 eggs
1 heaping cup (115 g) shredded Cheddar cheese
½ cup (36 g) broccoli florets, cut into very small pieces
½ teaspoon ground mustard
½ teaspoon garlic powder
½ teaspoon salt
¼ teaspoon onion powder
¼ teaspoon ground black pepper

Preheat the oven to 350°F (180°C) and coat a mini muffin tin with cooking spray. In a large bowl, mix the quinoa, eggs, cheese, broccoli, mustard, garlic powder, salt, onion powder, and pepper until combined. Divide the mixture evenly among the muffin cups, placing about 1 tablespoon (12 g) in each. Press down on each bite firmly with the back of a spoon. Bake for 20 minutes. Remove immediately from the pan and set on a cooling rack. Serve warm. Store leftovers in the refrigerator in a lidded container.

Yield: 2 dozen bites

"TRY IT" TIP

Quinoa acts as a binding agent. To get your kids used to the flavor of quinoa, try subbing cooked quinoa for breadcrumbs when making meatballs and meatloaf.

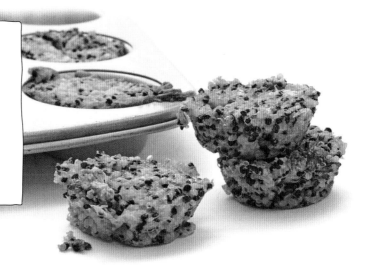

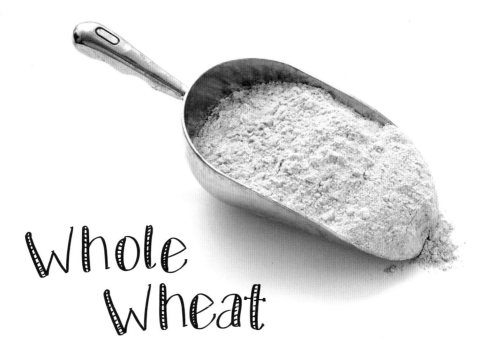

Whole Wheat

Most kids get plenty of wheat. It's in everything from crackers and cookies to bread and pasta and ranks as the most consumed grain in the country. But unfortunately, the most commonly eaten wheat is refined. That means it's been stripped of its bran and germ during processing to make it lighter in color and milder in flavor. That also takes away a lot of wheat's natural health benefits, such as fiber and vitamins (by law, refined flour must be enriched with some of the nutrients taken out during processing).

Whole wheat flour, which contains all parts of the wheat kernel, has **more protein, fiber, and vitamin E than refined flour**. For example, a serving of white pasta contains two grams of fiber, while the same portion of whole wheat packs five. Foods made with whole wheat also tend to be more filling and satisfying, likely due to the fiber. Whole wheat foods are associated with a **lower risk for type 2 diabetes, heart disease, and asthma** and **linked to a healthy body weight** too.

To find truly whole wheat products, be sure "whole wheat" is listed on the food's ingredient list. "Enriched flour" or "wheat flour" are both refined flours. When buying bagged flour, look for the words "whole wheat flour." Keep in mind that using whole wheat flour tends to result in heavier, denser baked goods. So try subbing it for one-quarter or one-half of the all-purpose flour in recipes. If you want to use all whole wheat flour, look for a recipe specifi-cally made for that. And take heart: In a study of elementary school children published in *Public Health Nutrition,* kids ate just as much pizza when it was made with a whole grain crust as they did when it was made with refined grains. Kids reported liking it just as much too.

Homemade Tortillas

Skip the store-bought kind with preservatives and added sugars. These tortillas go "halfsies" with all-purpose and whole wheat flour, plus just a few simple ingredients. The dough is easy enough for kids to roll out themselves.

1 cup (120 g) white whole wheat flour (or regular whole wheat flour), plus more for kneading the dough
1 cup (125 g) all-purpose flour
1 teaspoon baking powder
½ teaspoon salt
¼ cup (60 ml) olive oil
⅔ cup (160 ml) very warm water

In a medium bowl, mix the flours, baking powder, and salt. Add the oil and half of the water, stirring to combine. Add more water slowly, stirring until the dough comes together (you may not use all the water). Turn the dough out onto a lightly floured surface and knead for a minute, or until it forms a cohesive ball. Cut the dough into eight equal(ish) pieces, cover with a clean towel, and let rest for 30 minutes.

Preheat a cast-iron skillet (or a nonstick skillet coated with cooking spray) over medium-high heat while you roll out the first ball into a round, roughly 7 to 8 inches (18 to 20 cm) across. Place the round in the pan and cook for about a minute, or until bubbly and browned on the bottom, then flip and cook the other side. Repeat with each dough ball. Cool and store in an airtight container. Keep in the refrigerator if you don't use them within two days.

Yield: 8 tortillas

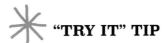 **"TRY IT" TIP**

If your kids are stuck on white pasta, try cooking up half white and half whole wheat. Then serve them together in one bowl and call it "Zebra Pasta." Likewise, use one slice each of white bread and whole wheat for sandwiches. Cut the sandwich into six pieces and flip three of them to create a checkerboard sandwich.

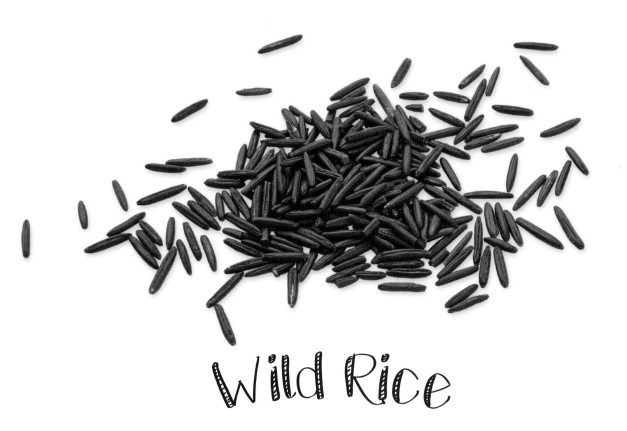

Wild Rice

If you want to raise more adventurous eaters, switching up the staples you regularly serve is key—like making different shapes of pasta or buying a wide variety of cheeses. If you frequently serve white or brown rice, wild rice makes for a fun change. It's still a familiar food (rice), but the color, texture, and even flavor are slightly different. Wild rice actually packs more nutrition too!

Wild rice is technically not a grain—it's a grass grown in lakes and rivers. It has been eaten for thousands of years and was a fixture in the diets of some Native American tribes. Today, Minnesota is the world's largest producer of wild rice. Because it's more difficult to grow than other varieties, it's more expensive. But you may be able to find it mixed with other kinds of rice and grains at an affordable price. It cooks up in just the same way as other rice does and "bursts" open when it's done.

Wild rice isn't refined during processing, so it's classified as a whole grain and has **three grams of fiber** (both soluble and insoluble) per cooked cup (164 g). It contains **more protein than brown or white rice**—with more than six grams per cup (that's about a third of what young kids need in a day!). And one study from the University of Manitoba found that the antioxidant activity of wild rice was thirty times higher than white. It's also **gluten free**. You can sub wild rice in recipes that call for brown or white rice. To add more fiber and plant protein to meat-based dishes, swap wild rice for part of the meat in meatloaf and burgers.

Q: Is Cereal Good for Kids?

Cereal is a prime source of nutrients such as iron and fiber for kids. But there are plenty of cereals on the market that seem more like dessert. Here's my quick-and-dirty guideline for choosing a cereal: Avoid varieties with artificial colors and flavors and pick a box with roughly five grams of sugar or fewer and at least three grams of fiber per serving. If your kids love sweetened cereal, mix a favorite sweet cereal with its unsweetened counterpart (such as sweetened Os mixed with unsweetened). Or buy an unsweetened cereal and add your own sweetness. Even if you sprinkle on a full teaspoon of sugar (or drizzle on a teaspoon of honey), it's still far less added sugar than you'd get with many boxed cereals.

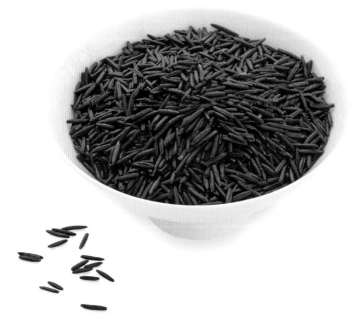

Good to Know

Any carbohydrate-rich food can be a cavity culprit—not just sticky candy. When foods such as crackers and cereal break down in the mouth, bacteria use them to make acid that can dissolve away tooth enamel. The risk is higher when kids nibble on these foods through-out the day, like many toddlers do! Be sure kids are brushing regularly and drinking water to help rinse their teeth. Apples and cheese are also natural tooth cleaners, so serving those foods with meals and snacks can help.

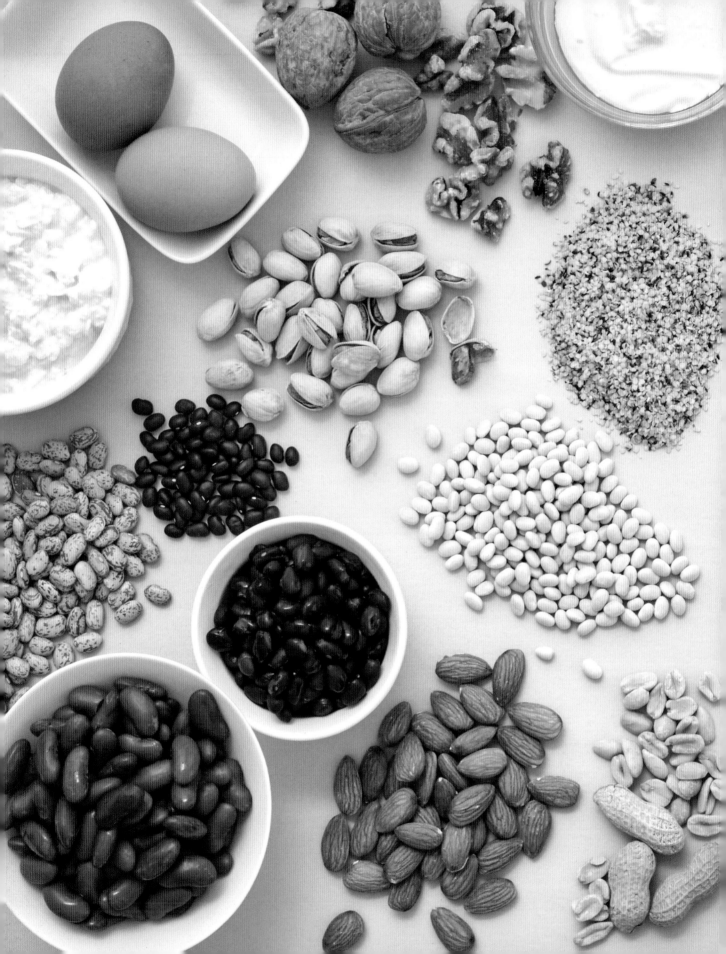

4

Protein-Rich Foods

PROTEIN IS THE NUTRIENT OF THE MOMENT, and it plays a starring role for kids during growth, building new cells and tissues, healing the body after stress or injury, repairing muscles after exercise, and providing energy to fuel the body. Protein is also an especially filling nutrient, making your child's meals and snacks more satisfying.

Yet for all the good that protein does for the body, it's also a source of stress for some parents, who worry their kids aren't getting enough—especially if they're hopelessly devoted to pasta (and not so much to meat). If you've got protein anxiety, I have good news. While meat, poultry, and fish are stellar sources of protein, it's abundant in a lot of other foods too—many of which your child probably already loves. And though this chapter is a collection of especially protein-rich picks, your kid is also nabbing protein throughout the day from foods in the grain and vegetable chapters too. In fact, it's not as hard as you might think for kids to meet their daily protein needs: A small peanut butter sandwich, a glass of milk, a half cup (80 g) of cooked peas, and a half cup (70 g) of pasta sprinkled with cheese supply more than enough for an eight-year-old.

HOW MUCH PROTEIN DOES YOUR KIDS NEED EVERY DAY?

These numbers are based on the Recommended Dietary Allowances (RDAs), which are the minimum amounts needed to meet your child's basic needs.

- Ages 1–3: 13 grams
- Ages 4–8: 19 grams
- Ages 9–13: 34 grams
- Ages 14–18: 46 grams (girls), 52 grams (boys)

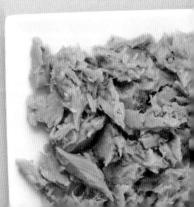

Beans

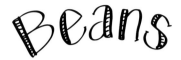

They're the "magical fruit" in the popular and giggle-inducing kids' rhyme, and I won't argue with that label (though technically, they're classified as both a veggie and a protein food by the USDA, not a fruit). Dry beans—such as black, kidney, navy, and pinto—are all **excellent, sustainable sources of plant protein**. Beans don't provide a "complete" protein like the kind found in meat—that means beans don't have all the amino acids (the building blocks of protein) that must be consumed through food. But eating beans and grains together in the same meal or simply in the same day can provide what the body needs.

Beans are also **a standout source of fiber**, including both soluble fiber (which helps reduce cholesterol levels and makes meals filling) and insoluble (which keeps the digestive system moving smoothly). A half cup of black beans contains seven grams of fiber—that's a third of what kids need in the entire day and something most kids don't get enough of. Beans are also a **great source of iron**, a mineral that's key during childhood for proper growth and development, and contain calcium, magnesium, zinc, and folate. Plus, dark-colored beans such as black beans pack anthocyanins, the same pigments found in grapes that work as antioxidants. Research has linked diets rich in beans to lower rates of heart disease and even a longer life.

And, yes, it's true, beans can also make you toot. Thanks to that fiber content, plus a starch that isn't broken down until it reaches the large intestine, eating beans can trigger gas production. Though it's likely more a source of hilarity to kids than an annoyance, you can help reduce the gas potential by rinsing canned beans before using them, discarding the water after soaking a batch of dry beans and using fresh water to cook them, and serving small portions at first if your kids aren't accustomed to eating so much fiber.

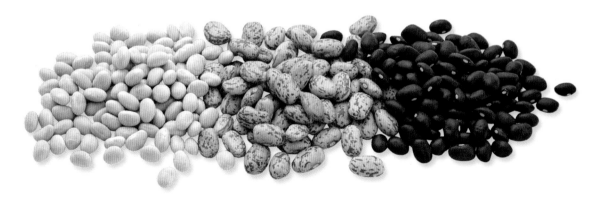

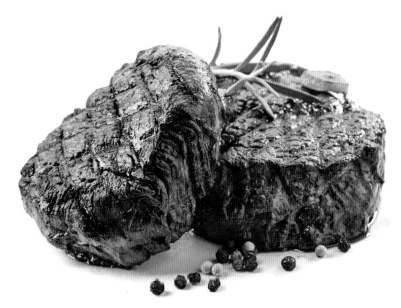

Beef

Beef doesn't sound like a first food for babies, but that's what many pediatricians now recommend. Old feeding advice advised introducing meat last, but the newest wisdom is to serve puréed meats such as beef early. The reason? Beef packs a hefty dose of both iron and zinc, and by six months, breast milk doesn't supply those nutrients in the amounts that babies need. Both are critical for growth and brain development; iron may have an impact on IQ, and zinc plays a role in reasoning and attention. Deficiencies during a child's early years can have devastating and lasting consequences on behavior and intelligence.

The nutrients in beef continue to be key for older kids too. A study published in the journal *Meat Science* found that lean beef consumption makes significant contributions to protein, iron, zinc, potassium, vitamin B_6, and vitamin B_{12} intakes among kids ages four to eighteen, and it didn't have a significant impact on total fat, saturated fat, or sodium intake. It's a **serious protein powerhouse**: Even a two-ounce (55 g) kid-sized portion packs as much protein as two cups (370 g) of quinoa or four tablespoons (65 g) of peanut butter. And **the iron it contains is highly "bioavailable"**—meaning it's easy for the body to take up and use the iron (compared to iron in plant foods, which isn't as easily used). If your kids don't like the chewy texture, ground beef and stewed meat may be more accepted.

"TRY IT" TIP

To boost nutrition, dice white button mushrooms and cook them with ground turkey or beef to make taco filling. Or mix chopped white button mushrooms with ground beef to make hamburger patties. They virtually disappear. Roast the mushrooms for ten to fifteen minutes before chopping to enhance their flavor.

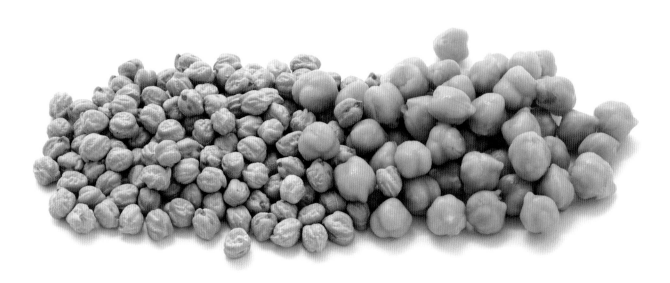

Chickpeas

Yes, they're technically beans. But they're so darn kid friendly that they deserve their own little spotlight. Also called garbanzo beans, chickpeas have been eaten since ancient times and are considered a "pulse" just like peas, lentils, and other beans. That means they boast all the same superstar health perks when you eat them regularly, including lower cholesterol and blood pressure levels and even a reduced risk of certain kinds of cancer.

Like all pulses, chickpeas are a **lean, healthy, and sustainable plant protein**. One-half cup (120 g) of chickpeas is loaded with **six grams of fiber** (a quarter of what kids need in the whole day) plus seven grams of protein (about as much as two slices of deli turkey). Chickpeas are also **packed with iron and zinc**, two minerals kids need as they're growing and developing, and a little bit of calcium and potassium.

You can buy dried chickpeas that you soak and cook yourself. Or opt for the convenience of canned ones. Chickpeas are a filling and respectable stand-in for meat if you're trying to serve more meatless meals, and they're good on top of a salad, added to soups, or in a curry. Newcomers may prefer to start with mashed chickpeas in hummus, served with lots of soft pita, or falafel, which is a traditional Middle Eastern "fritter" made from ground chickpeas that's typically deep-fried (but can be baked or pan-fried too).

Taco-Spiced Skillet Chickpeas

I convinced my thirteen-year-old, who swears up and down that he doesn't like chickpeas, to try one of these. Then he ate another. And another. And another. Why the sudden change of heart? His only explanation: "They taste like tacos!"

1 can (15 ounces [425 g]) chickpeas
½ teaspoon chili powder
½ teaspoon paprika
½ teaspoon ground cumin
¼ teaspoon garlic powder
¼ teaspoon onion powder
½ teaspoon salt
1 tablespoon (15 ml) olive oil

Drain and rinse the chickpeas, then pat dry with a paper towel or clean cloth, discarding any skins that come off. In a medium bowl, combine the chili powder, paprika, cumin, garlic powder, onion powder, and salt. In a skillet, heat the oil over medium heat for 30 seconds, then add the chickpeas, stirring and cooking until browned, 7 to 10 minutes. Remove from the heat, pour the chickpeas into the bowl with the seasoning, and toss well until covered. Serve immediately. Store leftovers in an airtight container in the refrigerator and pop them in the oven or toaster oven to reheat and add some crunch.

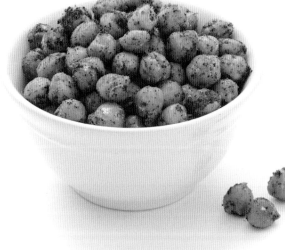

Yield: 2 to 4 servings

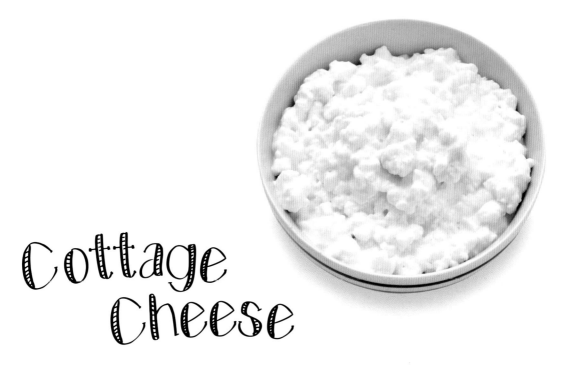

Cottage Cheese

You may still associate cottage cheese with leg warmer–clad dieters. But cottage cheese is worth a second look because it's **a good source of calcium for kids and rich in protein**. Childhood is a critical time to get calcium because the body is building new bone, a process that stops when we reach our twenties. Many children don't consume enough calcium, which could lead to low bone density and a higher risk for fractures as adults. Kids ages two to three need two servings of dairy a day, older kids three servings. One cup (225 g) of cottage cheese counts as a half serving.

Cottage cheese is made when the curds and whey in milk are separated, and the whey is removed. As with yogurt, even kids with lactose intolerance may be able to eat cottage cheese without a problem because of this. A half cup (115 g) of cottage cheese is **brimming with protein** (thirteen grams!), making it an even better source of high-quality protein than milk. It's also a **good source of calcium** for kids, plus vitamin B_{12}, riboflavin, phosphorus, and vitamin A. And the calcium in dairy products such as cottage cheese is typically easier for the body to absorb and use than the calcium in plant foods such as spinach. Cottage cheese can be eaten just like yogurt: Pair it with fresh fruit, or serve it swirled with some jam or honey.

HELP!
I Think My Child Is Lactose Intolerant!

People with lactose intolerance have trouble digesting the natural milk sugar in dairy called lactose. The lactose ends up being fermented in the colon, which can cause gas, bloating, belly pain, and diarrhea. (This is different from a milk allergy, which is an immune response and requires total avoidance of dairy.) If you suspect your child is lactose intolerant, talk to your pediatrician before self-diagnosing and cutting out all dairy, which is a helpful source of calcium, protein, and vitamin D for your child. Also, if your child is diagnosed, keep in mind that some people with lactose intolerance can consume small portions of dairy without having symptoms. Others can't tolerate milk but may be fine with yogurt and kefir. If your child doesn't tolerate any dairy, be sure to include alternative sources of calcium and vitamin D in her diet, such as fortified nondairy milks, cereal, and orange juice.

✳ "TRY IT" TIP

Familiarize your child with the flavor of cottage cheese by using it in place of ricotta (or subbing half of the ricotta) in lasagna and puréeing it to blend into the sauce for mac and cheese.

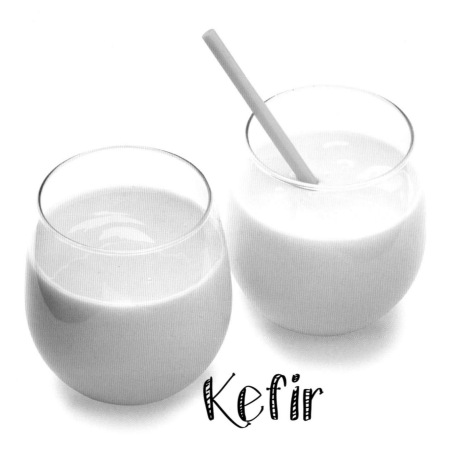

Kefir

If your kids already like the taste of store-bought drinkable yogurts, they'll probably like kefir too. (Just don't be like me and spend years calling it KEE-fer only to learn that it's actually pronounced kuh-FEAR.) Kefir is a fermented milk drink that's been enjoyed for thousands of years and hails from Western Asia. You'll find it in the dairy aisle or the natural foods refrigerated section of the grocery store. It's thick and tangy, and because the cultures used to ferment it also break down lactose, it ends up being largely lactose free. Some research has found that even people with lactose intolerance may be able to tolerate kefir (the same is not true of kids with milk allergy, who cannot have kefir or any product made with milk).

Like regular milk, kefir is an **excellent source of calcium and protein**. One cup (235 ml) contains 300 mg of bone-building calcium, about a third of what a four- to eight-year-old needs in a day, and eight grams of filling protein. Like milk, it may also be **fortified with vitamin D**, a mineral most kids and grown-ups are falling short on.

Because kefir is fermented, it's a **rich source of probiotics**, beneficial bacteria that populate the intestines and crowd out strains of harmful bacteria. Probiotics can help guard against stomach bugs and keep digestion running smoothly. Because many immune cells are located in the gut, probiotics are also thought to boost immunity and help fight off illness and infection.

Plain kefir is a bit sour but makes a thick, creamy base for smoothies. You can also find flavored kefir, which is much tastier to drink on its own and contains a couple teaspoons of added sugar for sweetness.

Good to Know

Probiotics work even better in the body when you include prebiotics in the diet too. Prebiotics "feed" the probiotics in the gut, helping them flourish. Food sources of prebiotics include bananas, onions, garlic, whole wheat, and asparagus. So try a combo like this. Make a smoothie with kefir and bananas, or a sandwich on whole wheat bread with a sour pickle on the side.

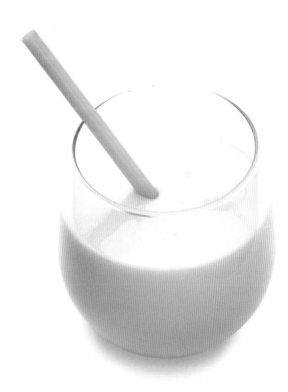

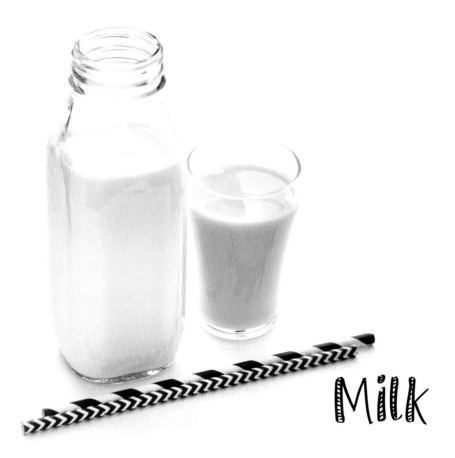

Milk

Milk is a **handy package of several key nutrients kids need**—such as calcium, magnesium, potassium, protein, and vitamin D—in one glass. No doubt, calcium is critical right now. Kids need to get enough while they're at their peak bone-building stage so they'll have strong skeletons going into adulthood. Kids ages four to eight need 1,000 mg of calcium per day, and that requirement jumps to 1,300 mg at age nine; serving milk with meals in a no-brainer way to get most of that calcium. Milk is also **fortified with vitamin D**, and many people (including kids) don't get enough of this vitamin because it's found in so few foods and drinks (sunscreen also blocks the rays that help our bodies naturally produce the vitamin).

If you're wondering what kind of milk to buy, keep in mind that all types (from full-fat to fat-free) have roughly the same amount of calcium, protein, vitamin D, and potassium. Concerns about saturated fat in dairy seem to be waning, and there's also some evidence, including a study published in the *American Journal of Clinical Nutrition,* that full-fat milk may be linked to a lower body mass index among kids (possibly because it's more filling than lower-fat milks). Unless your pediatrician tells you otherwise, serve whole milk to kids younger than age two because the fat is needed for brain development. Beyond age two, my advice is to stock the kind of milk your kids like and will reliably drink.

Does your child like only flavored milk? As a dietitian, I don't have a problem with flavored milk—as long as you and your child consider it a treat and balance out the sugar that day. Buy your own syrup or powder and control how much sweetness is added. Or combine half chocolate milk with half regular milk to keep the sweetness but lower the added sugar.

SOY MILK

Though new protein-fortified nut milks are appearing on shelves, soy milk is one of the few nondairy milks that is **naturally rich in protein**. One cup (235 ml) of soy milk contains eight grams of protein, the same as cow's milk. That's why calcium-fortified soy milk is the only nondairy milk to count as a serving of dairy in the USDA's MyPlate guidelines. Be sure the brand you buy is fortified with both calcium and vitamin D. It's been shown that the body can absorb calcium from soy products as well as it does from dairy. Just watch out for flavored soy milk, which can contain multiple teaspoons of added sugar per glass.

Good to Know

Be sure your toddler or preschooler isn't drinking too much milk. Excessive amounts of milk (more than three cups, or 720 ml, a day) can fill up their little bellies, so they may not be hungry for food at meals. That ups the risk for developing iron deficiency. Kids ages two to three need only two servings of dairy a day, kids ages four to eight should aim for 2½ servings, and kids nine and up need three. A serving of dairy is either a cup (235 ml) of milk or calcium-fortified soy milk, a cup (230 g) of yogurt, or 1½ ounces (43 g) of cheese.

Q: Is Raw Milk Safe for Kids?

While raw milk may have its legion of devoted fans, I think it's best to err on the side of safety. Raw milk isn't pasteurized to kill potentially harmful bacteria such as salmonella and *E. coli*, so there's a risk of infections that can lead to everything from diarrhea to life-threatening diseases. Babies and young children are among the groups most vulnerable to these raw milk risks. According to the Centers for Disease Control and Prevention, at least one child younger than five was involved in nearly 60 percent of the raw milk foodborne illness outbreaks reported from 2007 through 2012.

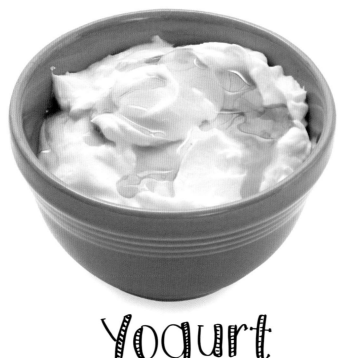

Yogurt

Yes, you'll find plenty of candy mix-ins, artificial flavors, and sweeteners in the yogurt aisle. But weed out the junk, and you'll find that plain yogurt is a healthy food that delivers a lot to your child's diet. Eaten for thousands of years, yogurt is milk that's been fermented by healthy bacteria. That bacteria does good things for us when we eat it, such as populating the digestive tract, where it crowds out unhealthy bacteria, helping **regulate digestion**, and even **supporting the immune system**. To make sure your family is getting the benefit, check the carton for a seal or a statement that the product contains "live and active cultures" (FYI: Frozen yogurt doesn't typically contain them!).

Some people who are lactose intolerant may even be able to eat yogurt without symptoms, thanks to the work the bacteria does of fermenting the milk's lactose (natural milk sugar) into lactic acid.

Rich in calcium and protein, yogurt does get a bad rap for being sugary—and some of that is deserved. There are many varieties that pack multiple teaspoons of added sugar per serving (even without those candy mix-ins!). But keep in mind that because of the natural lactose, even plain yogurt will list some sugar on the Nutrition Facts label. Plain yogurt contains about twelve grams of natural sugar per six ounces. (So a blueberry yogurt listing twenty-six grams of sugar has fourteen grams of added sugar—or about 3½ teaspoons.) Greek yogurt, which is made when the liquid whey is strained off during processing, is naturally lower in natural sugar and higher in protein than regular yogurt. It also has a thicker, creamier texture and a tangier taste.

Try buying plain yogurt and drizzle in your own honey or maple syrup. This helps reduce the tanginess that some kids don't love and also allows you to control how much extra sugar your child gets in her dish. Or mix half plain yogurt with half presweetened. It will still be sweet, but you'll cut the added sugar in half.

→ Very Berry Pops

These homemade berry pops, made with calcium-rich yogurt and whole fruit, rival the store-bought kind. At least my kids think so!

1 cup (250 g) frozen red raspberries
2 cups (460 g) vanilla yogurt
Juice and zest of ½ lemon

Place the raspberries in a small bowl and allow to defrost. Mash well with a fork and add the yogurt, lemon juice, and zest. Stir to combine. Pour into 4 small paper cups, leaving ½ inch (1 cm) of headspace. Cover the cups with plastic wrap and insert an ice pop stick through the wrap and into the pop. (Or pour into your favorite ice pop molds.) Freeze until hard, then peel away the paper.

Yield: 4 servings

Good to Know

Babies can have yogurt after they start solids around six months. Just choose a full-fat yogurt because babies need large amounts of fat in their diets for brain development. Opt for a plain variety too. Many babies actually delight in the flavor!

Edamame

The most kid-friendly form of soy may just be the bean itself! Edamame are whole green soybeans that have been steamed or boiled and then chilled. You'll typically find edamame in the frozen section of your grocery store, either shelled or unshelled (you eat only the beans inside, not the pod). The beans are firm, slightly sweet, and nutty, and sometimes they're lightly salted for extra flavor.

Edamame is an ideal snack for hungry kids because it's **loaded with two of the most filling nutrients**, protein and fiber. Just a half cup (78 g) of edamame in the pods contains five grams of high-quality protein (that's about a quarter of the protein young kids need in a day) and four grams of fiber. Soy is also a **rich source of iron**, and the iron from soy is actually better absorbed by the body than the iron found in many other plant-based foods. In addition, edamame is **a source of calcium, magnesium, and potassium**.

Pack a handful of the pods in your kids' lunch boxes, and they can squeeze the beans out of the pods and into their mouths with their fingers. Or serve them as a quick side for lunch or dinner (just a minute or less in the microwave, and the frozen pods are ready to serve). You can add the shelled beans to stir-fries and salads.

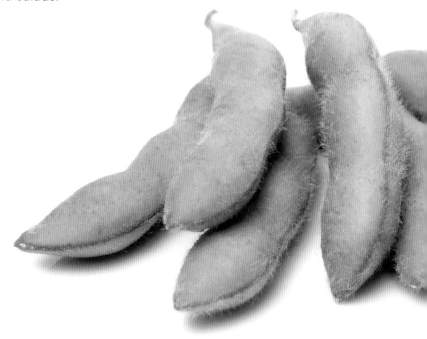

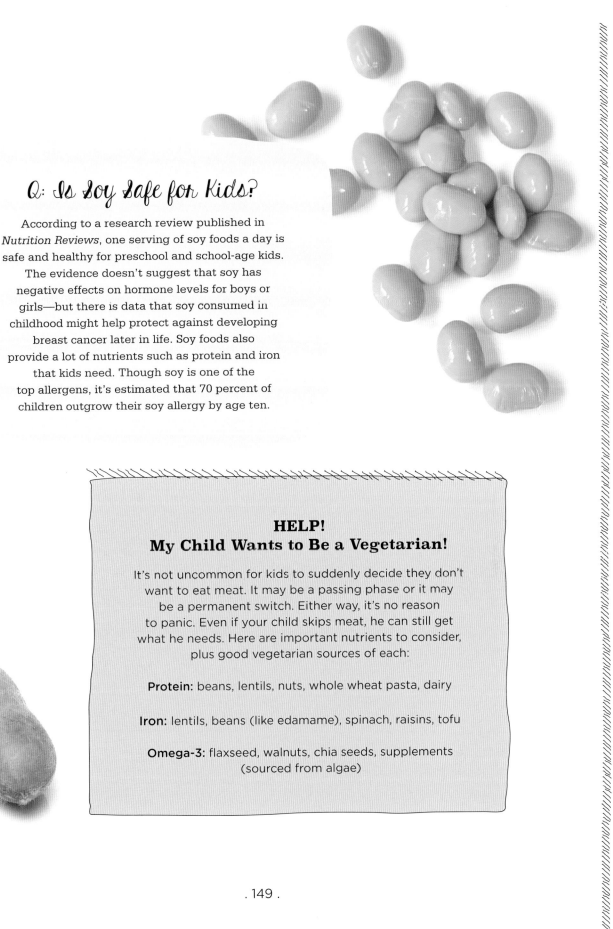

Q: Is Soy Safe for Kids?

According to a research review published in
Nutrition Reviews, one serving of soy foods a day is
safe and healthy for preschool and school-age kids.
The evidence doesn't suggest that soy has
negative effects on hormone levels for boys or
girls—but there is data that soy consumed in
childhood might help protect against developing
breast cancer later in life. Soy foods also
provide a lot of nutrients such as protein and iron
that kids need. Though soy is one of the
top allergens, it's estimated that 70 percent of
children outgrow their soy allergy by age ten.

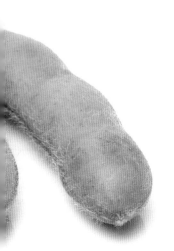

HELP!
My Child Wants to Be a Vegetarian!

It's not uncommon for kids to suddenly decide they don't
want to eat meat. It may be a passing phase or it may
be a permanent switch. Either way, it's no reason
to panic. Even if your child skips meat, he can still get
what he needs. Here are important nutrients to consider,
plus good vegetarian sources of each:

Protein: beans, lentils, nuts, whole wheat pasta, dairy

Iron: lentils, beans (like edamame), spinach, raisins, tofu

Omega-3: flaxseed, walnuts, chia seeds, supplements
(sourced from algae)

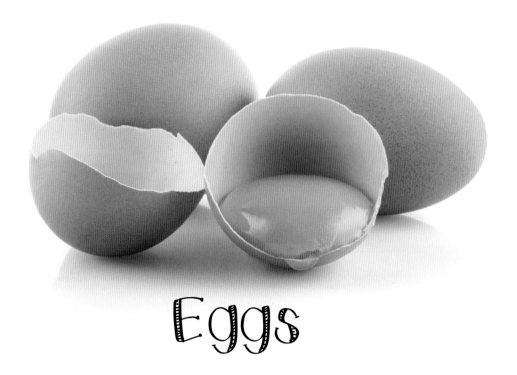

Eggs

Eggs are a small but mighty package of nutrients and a genuinely **affordable source of protein**. Even if you choose organic eggs, you'll spend less than fifty cents for a serving of high-quality protein. A **"high-quality" protein** means it has all nine essential amino acids, the kind the body doesn't make and you have to get through food. (Meat is also a high-quality protein, while most plants are missing at least one key amino acid.)

While the whites are a great source of protein, don't toss the yolk. It's loaded with valuable nutrients the whites don't have, including choline, a nutrient that helps transport vitamins and minerals around the body. Choline is vital during pregnancy for brain and spine development and continues to be critical for babies and young kids as their brains develop. The yolk is also **rich in lutein**, an antioxidant that's tied to brain function as well. In a study of children ages eight to nine published in *Nutritional Neuroscience*, a higher density of lutein in the brain (measured by a noninvasive eye test) was associated with higher academic achievement. There's also evidence that lutein may help protect the eye from "blue light" damage—that's the light emitted from the smartphones, tablets, and computers that are part of most kids' daily lives.

It's true that egg yolks are also naturally rich in cholesterol. But according to the Dietary Guidelines for Americans, evidence doesn't show that the cholesterol in foods such as eggs and shellfish drives up blood cholesterol levels. So even an egg every day is okay! Keep in mind that it's safe to keep eggs two to three weeks beyond the expiration date stamped on the carton.

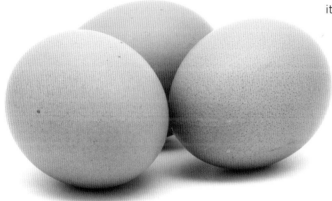

Good to Know

Hormones are never given to egg-laying hens, and they're banned from use in any poultry production. So if you spot "hormone free" on a package, it's simply marketing.

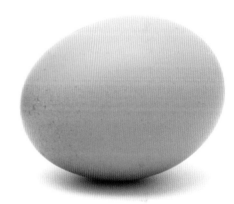

Q: Are Brown Eggs Healthier Than White?

Brown eggs may look more fresh and wholesome than white, but they're actually the same nutritionally. Brown eggs simply come from a different breed of chicken. So there's no need to pay more for them.

Lentils

A lot of families are looking to reduce their carbon footprint at the dinner table. If you count yourself among those, lentils should be your best friend. These little disk-shaped legumes are nutritional powerhouses yet a highly sustainable crop, drawing their own nitrogen from the air to use as fertilizer and requiring little water to grow. Lentils are considered a "pulse"—that's the edible seed of a plant in the legume family, and it includes foods such as dry peas, dry beans, and chickpeas. They've been eaten for more than 10,000 years (they're even name-checked in the famous Green poem *The Iliad* from the eighth century BCE!).

A one-half cup (99 g) serving of cooked green lentils has **nine grams of fiber,** more than half of what a young child needs in a day. Each half cup (99 g) also packs **12 grams of protein**—that's as much as a two-ounce (55 g) serving of beef. When lentils are eaten with a whole grain (such as lentils and brown rice), they form a complete protein, which means the meal provides all of the essential amino acids you need to get from food. They're also gluten free and **higher in folate**, a B vitamin linked to heart health, than any other plant food.

The most common kind of lentils you'll find in the store are whole green lentils and split red lentils. Split lentils have had their outer coating removed and are split in half (so they tend to cook more quickly but have less fiber and protein). You can buy lentils dried or canned—but unlike dry beans, there's no need to soak dry lentils before cooking. After a quick rinse, they cook in about 15 to 30 minutes.

Red Lentil Snack Cookies

If your kids aren't familiar with lentils, combining their new flavor and texture with old favorites such as peanut butter and chocolate chips in a lightly sweet and filling cookie may encourage them to try lentils in other ways.

½ cup (96 g) uncooked red lentils
½ cup (130 g) natural creamy peanut butter
1½ cups (234 g) old-fashioned oats
¼ cup (30 g) whole wheat flour
1 egg
½ cup (125 g) unsweetened applesauce
¼ cup plus 1 tablespoon (100 g) maple syrup
1 teaspoon vanilla extract
½ teaspoon baking soda
¼ teaspoon salt
¼ cup (44 g) chocolate chips

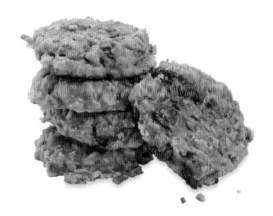

Rinse the lentils and place in a small saucepan. Cover with 1½ cups (360 ml) water and bring to a boil. Cover, reduce the heat, and simmer for 10 to 15 minutes, or until most of the water is absorbed and the lentils are soft. Transfer the lentils to a small colander to drain away excess liquid.

In the bowl of a food processor, combine the lentils, peanut butter, 1 cup (156 g) of the oats, the flour, egg, applesauce, maple syrup, vanilla, baking soda, and salt and process until well blended. Add the remaining ½ cup (78 g) of oats and the chocolate chips and pulse a few times just until incorporated. Cover the bowl and chill the mixture in the refrigerator for 30 minutes.

Preheat the oven to 375°F (190°C) and line a baking sheet with parchment paper or a silicone baking mat. Drop heaping tablespoons (15 g) of batter onto the baking sheet (a small cookie scoop is a great tool for this job). They won't spread, so don't worry about spacing them far apart. Gently press down the tops of the cookies with the bottom of a small glass or measuring cup dipped lightly in flour. Bake for 12 minutes. Remove to a cooling rack. Keep leftovers refrigerated in an airtight container.

Yield: about 2½ dozen cookies

Lentils (continued)

Good to Know

It's never too late to introduce kids to new foods. In a study with children ages three to six published in *Food Quality and Preference,* offering lentils one to two times per week for thirteen weeks increased both the children's liking and intake of lentils—even among kids who had never had them before.

 "TRY IT" TIP

Mix one part cooked lentils with two to three parts ground beef when making filling for sloppy joes or tacos. You can also blend cooked lentils (or beans) to make a quick veggie dip.

Q: Is Protein Powder Safe for Kids?

These powders may be all the rage, but in most cases, kids simply don't need the extra protein. Their protein requirements aren't very high and can usually be met pretty easily with food, even if they're vegetarian. Protein powders also tend to have a long list of ingredients and may include added sweeteners (real or artificial), flavorings, and other additives. Though some are billed as meal replacements, it's much healthier for your child (and better for her long-term habits) to eat actual food instead.

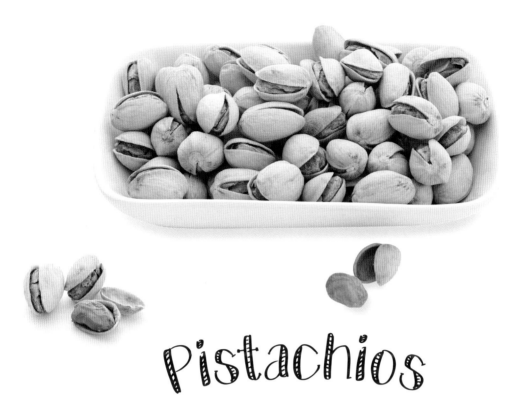

Pistachios

The fact is, all nuts are good for you—and because each one has slightly different health perks, there's no reason to favor one over another. But among commonly eaten tree nuts, pistachios have the honor of being **the richest in phytosterols**, according to a study in the *Journal of Agricultural and Food Chemistry.* Those are natural plant chemicals ("phyto" means "plant") that may help lower cholesterol levels. Pistachios also contain lutein, an antioxidant that can protect eyes from disease and from blue light (the kind emitted from cell phones and tablets). Plus, they are an **excellent source of iron** for kids and supply potassium for healthy blood pressure and phosphorus for healthy bones. And talk about a filling snack: A quarter cup (31 g) of shelled pistachio kernels is packed with **six grams of protein** and three grams of fiber, plus healthy (and satisfying) unsaturated fat.

Pistachios have been grown for thousands of years in the Middle East but are now cultivated in the United States too. They grow on trees in bunches like grapes and have tan shells with green kernels inside (if you've ever seen the nuts with red shells, that's a dye used on some imported pistachios to disguise imperfections!). Pistachios naturally crack open as they ripen, but if they're too tough for your kid to crack, look for bags of them already shelled. Besides snacking on them straight-up, you can also finely chop them for a breading on chicken and fish or add them to homemade pesto in place of walnuts.

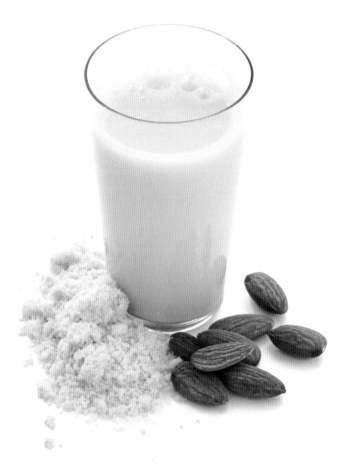

Almonds

Almonds are an overachiever, containing the most protein, fiber, calcium, vitamin E, riboflavin, and niacin of any tree nut. They're good for your child's heart, with **cholesterol-lowering fiber and healthy unsaturated fat** and **good for their bones**, with magnesium and a surprising amount of calcium that's easily absorbed by the body to help strengthen the skeleton (one ounce, or 28 g, of almonds has 75 mg of calcium; kids ages four to eight need 1,000 mg of calcium per day). Almonds are also **one of the richest food sources of vitamin E**, which works as an antioxidant in the body to squash free radicals that can damage cells and DNA.

They're good for the gut, with fiber to help stave off constipation—and some research shows that almonds may also act as a prebiotic in the digestive system, nourishing the healthy bacteria so it can thrive. In a study published in the journal *Nutrition Research,* kids and parents who had almonds or almond butter every day improved the overall quality of their diets and had healthy changes occur in their gut bacteria. Bonus: They didn't

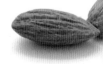

end up taking in more calories overall, likely because nuts are so filling. In fact, even though nuts and nut butters are calorie dense, research shows that regular consumption of almonds doesn't lead to weight gain and isn't associated with having a higher body mass index.

You can add slivered almonds to your child's oatmeal or granola, use almond butter in place of peanut butter, or bake with almond flour if your child eats a gluten-free diet. Almond milk is handy for smoothies, but keep in mind that even though almonds are high in protein, almond milk is not. In fact, there's only one gram per serving. That's important to know if you're swapping it for regular cow's milk (which has eight grams of protein per cup, or 235 ml).

Good to Know

Whole nuts and globs of nut butter should never be given to children younger than four because they're choking hazards.

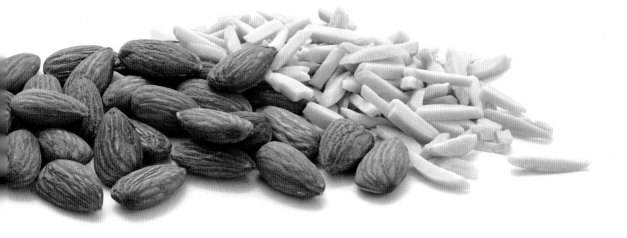

Peanuts

The humble peanut doesn't get nearly enough credit. Almonds and walnuts may steal all the accolades as superfood nuts, but peanuts boast just as many health benefits. Plus, they are economical, costing up to half as much as tree nuts. That's probably why peanuts make up about two-thirds of the nut consumption in the United States.

Even though they're technically legumes, peanuts are **heart healthy** just like tree nuts. They're rich in monounsaturated fats, which can help lower "bad" LDL cholesterol. They're also **high in fiber**. Each ounce (28 g, or roughly the amount you can fit in your palm in a single layer) has nearly three grams—and whole peanuts in the shell, which still have their skins, deliver even more. They're also **the highest-protein nut**, with nearly eight grams (the same amount as a glass of milk) per ounce. That package of filling nutrients makes peanuts and peanut butter especially satisfying, and when meals and snacks are filling, there's less chance of overeating. In fact, research finds that kids who eat peanuts and peanut butter have lower body mass indexes (BMIs) than those who don't, and a 2007 study published in *Pediatrics* found that twelve-year-olds who substituted peanuts or peanut butter for an unhealthy snack every day after school improved their weight status and nutrient intake. When selecting nut butter, look for "natural" varieties and ingredient lists that include just nuts (or nuts and salt).

Though the old advice was to hold off on peanuts until age three because of potential allergies, peanut protein has now been deemed safe and even beneficial for babies. The latest guidelines say that babies who are at high risk for peanut allergy due to eczema or egg allergy should be exposed to peanut protein (typically in the form of peanut powder mixed into their food) as young as four to six months when they start solids. Babies with mild to moderate eczema should be introduced to it by six months. Other babies can have it any time after starting solids. Always talk to your pediatrician about when to introduce it. Your baby may require an allergy test first, and you may be advised to give the first feeding under medical supervision.

Homemade Peanut Butter

Fresh peanut butter straight out of the food processor is a real treat!

2 cups (290 g) roasted peanuts (salted or unsalted)
Optional add-ins: pinch of salt, drizzle of honey, few squares chocolate

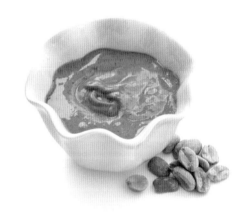

Place the peanuts in the bowl of a food processor and let it run. First the peanuts will appear dry and crumbly, then moist like wet sand. Then the mixture will appear doughy and may form a ball that will bang around the bowl. Finally, the peanuts will release their oils, and the mixture will become smooth. At this time, you can add salt (if using unsalted peanuts), honey, or chocolate—or keep it plain. Remove from the food processor. Store in a jar with a lid, and keep in the pantry if using within a week. Otherwise, store in the refrigerator. If oil rises to the top, simply stir it back in.

Yield: About 1 cup (250 g)

Good to Know

Even salted peanuts are considered a low-sodium food: One ounce (28 g) has just 90 mg of sodium, less than a typical bowl of cereal!

✳ "TRY IT" TIP

Serve peanut butter as a dip with veggies. In a study published in the *Journal of the American Dietetic Association,* kids who were served raw celery, broccoli, and carrots with peanut butter for dipping over the course of four weeks ate more veggies (and a greater variety of veggies) by the end of the study period than those served the vegetables without dip.

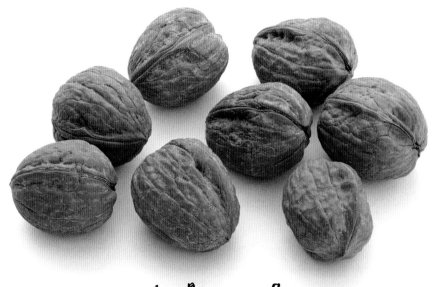

Walnuts

Walnuts earn a shout-out because they have **the most omega-3 fats** of all nuts. Walnuts contain a plant-based form of omega-3s called alpha-linolenic acid (ALA), the same kind found in flaxseed. Those are different from the omega-3s found in fish (EPA and DHA), which may help reduce risk for heart disease and are good for the brain and eyes. Though there's not as much evidence yet about ALA's heart-health perks, they're thought to help reduce inflammation in the body, which in turn can help reduce risk of some disease. ALA is also considered an essential fatty acid (meaning we have to get it from food), and a small amount of the ALA we consume converts to EPA in the body. A one-ounce (28 g) serving of walnuts has more than twice the amount of ALA kids need in a whole day. That same serving (about a quarter cup, or 28 g) also has two grams of fiber and **four grams of protein,** and it's an **excellent source of vitamin B$_6$** and the minerals copper, phosphorus, and magnesium. Walnuts also contain some iron and a little bit of calcium.

Walnuts stay fresher when they're kept cold, so stash them in the refrigerator once you've opened the package if you're planning to use them within a month (keep them away from strong-smelling items such as fish, since the walnuts can absorb the odors). Otherwise, tuck them into the freezer. Soaking walnuts for at least one to two hours (or up to overnight) can reduce their bitterness and bring out a richer flavor. Then you can blend them into smoothies for extra fiber, protein, and heft. Or chop them to add to oatmeal or the batter for pancakes and waffles. Finely chopped walnuts can also be used as a binder in meatballs and a coating for chicken and fish. I like roasting and chopping walnuts to add to pasta in place of meat.

Good to Know

Thanks to tannins, walnuts can taste slightly bitter, but roasting will help tame some of that flavor. Here's how: Place walnut halves on a baking sheet and bake at 350°F (180°C) for 8 to 10 minutes, or until lightly browned, shaking the pan halfway through the cooking time. Then chop and add into your recipe.

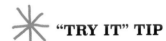 **"TRY IT" TIP**

In a food processor, pulse walnuts and cauliflower (or mushrooms) and add to taco meat or pasta sauces in place of some (or all) of the meat.

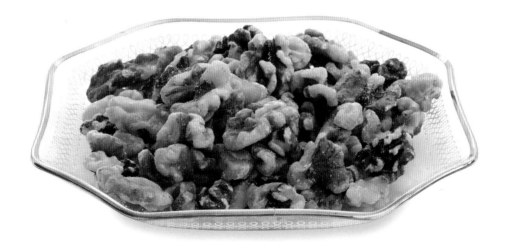

Chia Seeds

Remember the as-seen-on-TV Chia Pet that magically sprouted "fur"? The tiny black seeds that made it happen are actually good to eat—and really good for you. In fact, two tablespoons (24 g) have **nearly ten grams of fiber**. That's 40 percent of what kids need every day! The seeds are also a **good source of iron** and contain protein too. Because they're so rich in fiber, they are filling and can make meals and snacks more satisfying.

Another reason chia seeds have earned a superfood status: They **contain omega-3 fats**, which are known for their heart-health benefits. The omega-3s in chia seeds (and other foods such as flaxseed and walnuts) are called ALAs and are different from the omega-3 fats called EPA and DHA found in fish. But there is some evidence ALA may have positive effects on cholesterol and blood pressure too. Plus, a small amount of the ALA that's eaten is converted to EPA and DHA in the body.

So you've bought a bag—now what? You can toss chia seeds into home-made granola, baked goods, and breading for fish and chicken for extra crunch. Chia seeds also do something your kids will think is super-cool: They soak up liquid and become a gel. Try making a chia pudding by mixing them with almond milk and other add-ins such as cinnamon or vanilla, or combine them with puréed fruit to make your own quick jam. Unlike with flaxseed, you don't have to grind them up to get all the nutrients (though you can also buy ground chia seeds if you like that texture better). Stash them in the refrigerator or freezer to keep them fresh.

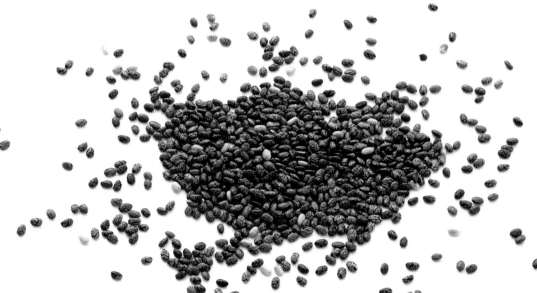

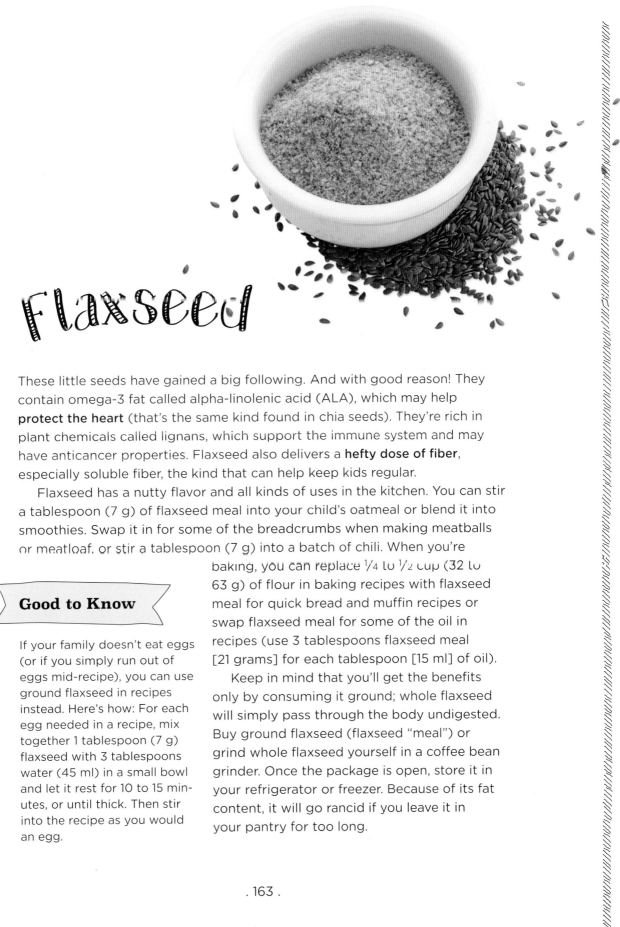

Flaxseed

These little seeds have gained a big following. And with good reason! They contain omega-3 fat called alpha-linolenic acid (ALA), which may help **protect the heart** (that's the same kind found in chia seeds). They're rich in plant chemicals called lignans, which support the immune system and may have anticancer properties. Flaxseed also delivers a **hefty dose of fiber**, especially soluble fiber, the kind that can help keep kids regular.

Flaxseed has a nutty flavor and all kinds of uses in the kitchen. You can stir a tablespoon (7 g) of flaxseed meal into your child's oatmeal or blend it into smoothies. Swap it in for some of the breadcrumbs when making meatballs or meatloaf, or stir a tablespoon (7 g) into a batch of chili. When you're baking, you can replace ¼ to ½ cup (32 to 63 g) of flour in baking recipes with flaxseed meal for quick bread and muffin recipes or swap flaxseed meal for some of the oil in recipes (use 3 tablespoons flaxseed meal [21 grams] for each tablespoon [15 ml] of oil).

Keep in mind that you'll get the benefits only by consuming it ground; whole flaxseed will simply pass through the body undigested. Buy ground flaxseed (flaxseed "meal") or grind whole flaxseed yourself in a coffee bean grinder. Once the package is open, store it in your refrigerator or freezer. Because of its fat content, it will go rancid if you leave it in your pantry for too long.

Good to Know

If your family doesn't eat eggs (or if you simply run out of eggs mid-recipe), you can use ground flaxseed in recipes instead. Here's how: For each egg needed in a recipe, mix together 1 tablespoon (7 g) flaxseed with 3 tablespoons water (45 ml) in a small bowl and let it rest for 10 to 15 minutes, or until thick. Then stir into the recipe as you would an egg.

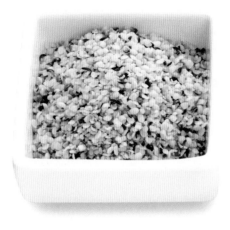
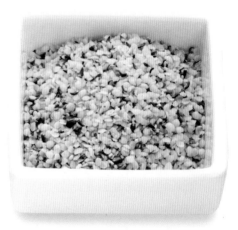

Hemp Seeds

First things first: While hemp seeds do come from the same plant species as marijuana, they don't contain the same active compound, so there's no danger to anyone, including kids, from consuming them (and nobody will test positive on a drug test after eating them!). Hemp seeds come from the hemp plant, which is a different crop than the marijuana plant and is also used to make goods such as paper and fabric.

These tiny seeds have a nutty flavor and a tender texture, and they're packed with nutrients that kids need. Each tablespoon (7 g) has **three grams of satisfying protein** plus a gram of fiber. They're a **stellar source of iron**, which carries oxygen to cells, and magnesium, which helps the body produce energy. They also contain phosphorus for healthy bones as well as zinc, a vital mineral for growth. In addition, hemp seeds provide **heart-protective omega-3 fatty acids** and a unique omega-6 fatty acid called gamma-linolenic acid (GLA) that may act as an anti-inflammatory (inflammation is believed to be linked to chronic disease).

You'll find bags of hemp seeds already shelled (hemp "hearts"), and you can sprinkle them right onto yogurt, oatmeal, cereal, or even grilled vegetables to add some texture and flavor. You can also add them to homemade granola and snack balls and bars.

Q: Are Dairy-Free Milks a Good Choice?

They can be. Some kids can't drink regular dairy milk because of an intolerance or allergy or because the family follows a vegan diet. Nondairy milks can be a nutritious replacement, but they aren't one-for-one swaps, nutritionally. Most nondairy milks such as rice and almond are actually very poor sources of protein. To get a comparable amount of protein to dairy milk (about eight grams per glass), you'll want to choose soy milk, pea protein milk, or protein-fortified nondairy milks. Keep in mind that some nondairy milks are also sweetened and contain multiple teaspoons of added sugar per glass, so check labels when buying them. One more caution: Homemade nondairy milks such as almond and cashew aren't good sources of calcium and vitamin D; store-bought versions of these milks are fortified with those nutrients.

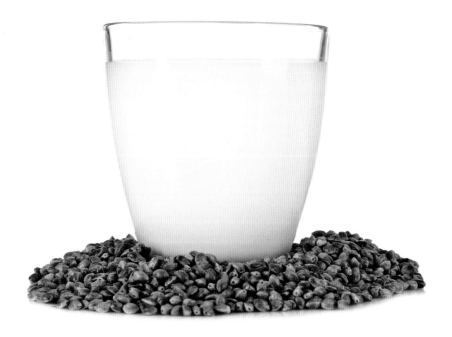

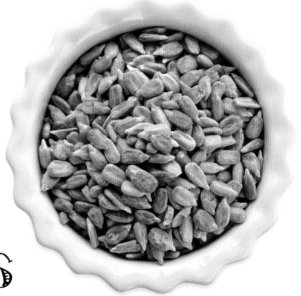

Sunflower Seeds

They're a mainstay of birdseed mixes and a fixture in baseball dugouts, but sunflower seeds are also an affordable superfood. Researchers ranked them tops among commonly eaten seeds in phytosterol content. Those are plant chemicals that can naturally block some cholesterol from being absorbed and lower cholesterol levels in the blood, which is good for heart health. They're also **loaded with vitamin E**, which works as an antioxidant in the body and may help prevent the kind of plaque buildup in the arteries that leads to heart disease. Plus, they're a **good source of selenium**, a mineral that also acts as a cell-protective antioxidant and is being studied for a possible role in cancer prevention too.

One-quarter cup (36 g) of sunflower kernels—the "meat" inside the hull—contains seven grams of protein (nearly as much as a glass of milk) and three grams of fiber, so they're a **satisfying snack** or mix-in to granola, muffins, oatmeal, and quick breads. (We eat them on green salads in lieu of croutons!) Nuts and seeds are rich in fat, but the majority of the fat is the healthy mono-unsaturated and polyunsaturated kind. A rich source of iron, the seeds provide minerals including potassium, magnesium, and phosphorus.

If your child is allergic to peanuts or tree nuts (or you need lunch box ideas for a nut-free cafeteria), look for sunflower seed butter. Made from sunflower seeds, it's a great source of protein and minerals such as iron and zinc. You can use it just as you would peanut butter. Just always check labels to be sure the brand you choose is peanut and nut free and not made in a facility with peanuts or tree nuts.

Nut-Free Snack Balls

Most snack ball recipes call for nuts or nut butter—and a food processor for blending. This one is not only nut and peanut free but can also be stirred together in a bowl. Remember to check labels on all ingredients if you need to avoid nuts and peanuts (and feel free to substitute peanut or almond butter for the sunflower seed butter if allergies aren't a concern).

¾ cup (60 g) quick oats
½ cup (130 g) sunflower seed butter
½ cup (14 g) crisped rice cereal (use brown crisped rice cereal if you can find it)
3 tablespoons (60 g) honey
1 tablespoon (7 g) ground flaxseed
⅓ cup (59 g) chocolate chips (optional, for coating)

In a small bowl, combine the oats, sunflower seed butter, rice cereal, honey, and flaxseed and mix until incorporated. Roll tablespoon-size (15 g) portions into balls. If the mixture is too sticky, add a bit more cereal or oats. If it's too dry, add a bit more sunflower seed butter. Place on a plate lined with parchment paper and freeze for at least 30 minutes. Store in the freezer or refrigerator. Optional: In the microwave, melt the chocolate chips in a small bowl, heating for 30-second intervals and stirring until melted. Using a spoon, dip one end of each snack ball into the melted chocolate and place on a parchment lined plate. Place in the freezer until the chocolate sets, then transfer to an airtight container in the refrigerator.

Yield: About 15 balls

Good to Know

Though the hull of sunflower seeds is edible (it's mostly fiber), there have been documented cases of children becoming severely constipated due to sunflower seeds becoming impacted in the large intestine. So have your kids spit out the hulls (baseball-player style) or buy them already shelled as kernels.

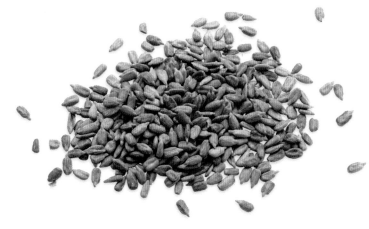

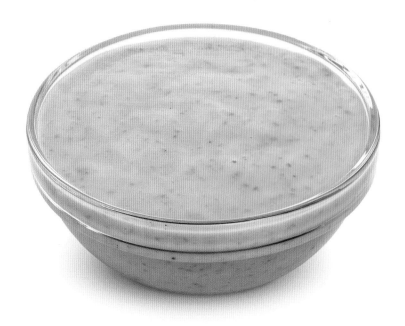

Tahini

Tahini is what transforms puréed chickpeas into hummus and roasted eggplant into baba ghanoush. This staple of Middle Eastern cooking is a paste made from ground roasted sesame seeds. Sesame seeds, which are probably best known for studding hamburger buns and bagels, are actually loaded with nutrition, including protein, fiber, and minerals such as copper and magnesium. They contain plant chemicals called lignans that may be **natural cancer fighters**, and like sunflower seeds, they're also high in phytosterols that **help lower cholesterol**. One tablespoon (15 g) of tahini has three grams of protein, a **hefty dose of iron**, plus fiber and calcium.

Look for tahini in the ethnic foods or natural foods aisle of the grocery store. Here are some labels you might see: "Hulled" tahini means the outer coating of the sesame seeds was removed to make a creamier spread ("unhulled" has more fiber but may be slightly more bitter). "Roasted" tahini will have a nuttier flavor than "raw."

The texture is similar to natural nut butters like peanut or almond—and like those butters, tahini tends to separate, so just stir it well before using to reincorporate the oil. Then store it in the refrigerator once opened so it doesn't go rancid. If you're feeling ambitious, you can make your own tahini by toasting raw sesame seeds on the stovetop or in the oven and grinding them in a food processor along with some mild-tasting oil such as light olive. Beyond blending it into dips and spreads, you can also use tahini to make a creamy salad dressing, stir a dollop into a heart stew or curry, or swap it for nut butter in cookies and other baked goods.

Easy Peasy Hummus

You're just a few minutes away from a batch of homemade hummus. This one has plenty of zing from fresh lemon. Serve it alongside carrot sticks, cucumber slices, and wedges of whole wheat pita bread.

2 cans (15.5-ounce/439 g) chickpeas, drained (reserve the liquid)
Juice of 2 lemons
1 large clove garlic
3 tablespoons (45 ml) tahini
1 teaspoon salt
Ground black pepper, to taste
¼ cup (60 ml) olive oil

Place the chickpeas, lemon juice, garlic, tahini, salt, and pepper in a blender or food processor and blend.

With the blender or food processor running, drizzle in the olive oil.

Stop the machine and scrape the sides. Then continue to blend, drizzling in the reserved liquid from the beans until you get the consistency you want.

Store in the refrigerator in an airtight container.

Yield: About 3 cups (738 g)

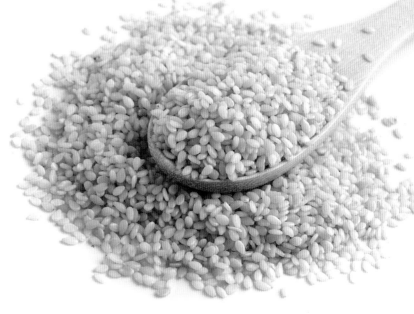

Salmon

There are many varieties of fish that are healthy choices, so why does salmon grab so much of the spotlight? Salmon is unique because unlike some popular fish varieties such as tilapia, it is an oily fish and contains a greater amount of the long-chain omega-3 fatty acids eicosapentaenoic acid (EPA) and docosahexaenoic acid (DHA). These fatty acids are so valuable because the body can't make them (we have to get them from food) and they protect the heart by doing a few things: They help thin the blood, which helps prevent the clots that can cause heart attacks and strokes. They also help prevent the arteries from hardening, which can lead to heart disease, and help lower triglycerides, a kind of fat in the blood.

You can also consider DHA to be **brain food for your kids**. It's the main omega-3 fat located in the brain's gray matter, where it may play a role in functions such as memory, attention, and even mood. Research has found that DHA taken during pregnancy and infancy is associated with higher IQs for children by preschool. And a deficiency in omega-3s has been identified in children with problems such as ADHD and dyslexia. DHA is also located in the eyes, where it may help **maintain healthy vision**. Some research has found that babies with higher levels of DHA in their blood have sharper vision. Like all fish, salmon is also **rich in protein and iron**.

If you've shopped for salmon, you've probably wondered whether wild-caught or farmed salmon is the better choice. Wild-caught has an edge, thanks to lower levels of contaminants. But farmed, which

Good to Know

When serving salads at dinner, skip fat-free dressing. Research shows that your body will better absorb the veggies' carotenoids, which are beneficial plant pigments, when they're paired with healthy fats, so use a full-fat salad dressing. Alongside salmon, it's a healthy meal!

Babies *can* eat fish! And they should, because the omega-3 fats found in fish are especially good for their developing brains. Pediatricians now give the green light to feeding fish to babies any time after six months when they're starting solids, so start with puréed fish and progress to well-mashed (making sure there are no bones left behind). If you have a family history of food allergies or have concerns, talk to your child's pediatrician before introducing it.

may have slightly higher levels of omega-3 (and tends to be less expensive), is a fine alternative. My advice is simply to serve the salmon that's available and affordable to you and to vary the kinds of fish you buy. The American Heart Association says that kids should eat fish twice a week to reap the benefits.

 "TRY IT" TIP

Sweeten the deal. I won my younger son over by brushing barbecue sauce onto salmon fillets before baking. The sweet, familiar flavor got him hooked!

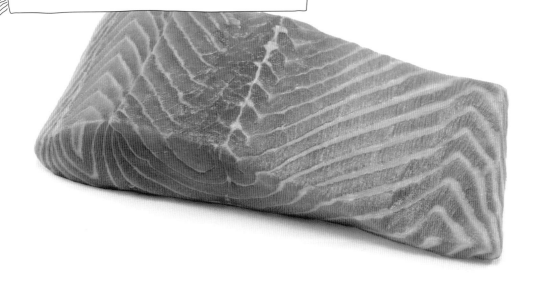

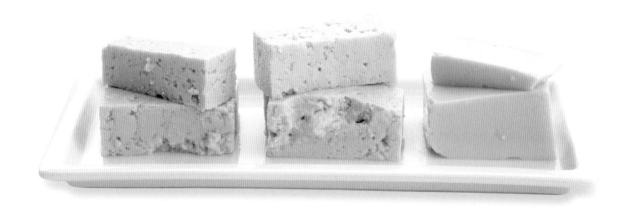

Tofu

Tofu can be a hard sell for some kids. Straight-up, it's not much to look at—and it doesn't taste like much either. It's also a little rubbery, and you won't find many picky eaters clamoring to try "coagulated soybean protein." But tofu has two key superpowers: It soaks up whatever flavor it's given like a champ. It can also take on many forms, from fried "meaty" pieces to a smooth sauce.

Tofu is made from soybean curds in a process similar to how cheese is created. It's sold in blocks, packed in water, in a few different varieties: Silken tofu (the softest kind) is perfect for blending into smoothies, sauces, and desserts for a protein boost. Firm tofu is best for baking. Extra-firm is hefty enough to stand up to stir-fries and kebabs.

Tofu is a worthy addition to a kid's diet because it's a **high-quality protein**, with all nine essential amino acids the body needs to get from food. That's tough to get in a plant food! Soy protein **may also help lower "bad" LDL cholesterol levels**. If your kids are turned off by the texture, choose extra-firm tofu and press out the excess liquid. Here's how: Place the block of tofu on a clean dish towel or paper towel on a plate. Cover it with another towel, and place something heavy (such as a cast-iron skillet) on top. I usually prop up one side of the plate so the liquid can drain to the other side and be poured away easily. To drain away even more water, slice your tofu into smaller pieces before pressing.

Speedy Miso Noodle Soup

Got ramen fans in the house? Toss the seasoning packet in the trash and make your own homemade batch quickly and easily. This recipe uses miso, a fermented paste made from soybeans and grain that lends a rich, savory flavor to broth. If your kids won't like the green onion or carrot, simply omit it from their bowls.

1 package (3 ounces [85 g]) ramen-style soup
1 cup (235 ml) water
1 cup (235 ml) low-sodium chicken or vegetable broth
1 tablespoon (16 g) white miso paste
1 teaspoon soy sauce
¼ cup (62 g) extra-firm tofu, cut into ½-inch (1 cm) cubes
¼ cup (28 g) shredded carrots
1 green onion, sliced into small rounds (green end only)

Open the package of ramen noodles and discard the seasoning packet. Cook the noodles in boiling water, drain, and set aside. In a small saucepan, heat the water and broth over medium heat. Add the miso paste and soy sauce and whisk until combined, stirring and heating until the mixture comes to a boil. Remove from the heat and stir in the tofu, carrots, and green onion. Divide between 2 bowls and serve.

Yield: 2 servings

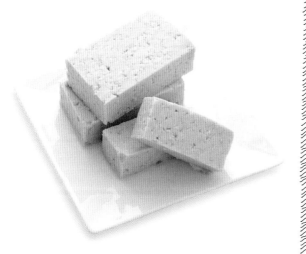

✳ "TRY IT" TIP

For tofu newbies, the crisper the better. If you don't want to deep-fry it, cut tofu in small pieces and bake them for about 30 minutes at 400°F (200°C), turning the pieces once. Then add them to a skillet, along with a tiny bit of oil, and lightly pan-fry them until the edges are crisp. Remove from the skillet and toss with Easy Peanut Sauce (see page 183).

Tuna

If you're wowed by the health benefits of fish (and you should be!), but you have sticker shock at the store's seafood counter, then consider tuna. Canned and pouch tuna is one of the most economical ways to fit fish into the diet, and you can't beat the convenience. The American Heart Association says that kids should eat fish twice a week because it's rich in high-quality protein, iron, and omega-3 fats without much saturated fat. Two ounces (55 g) of tuna has a whopping **ten grams of protein** and is a **good source of iron**, vitamin B_{12}, and niacin too. Tuna is also a source of omega-3 fatty acids, a kind of healthy fat found in some fish that's **good for kids' hearts and developing brains**. It's true that canned tuna has faced some scrutiny about its mercury content. You can lessen your child's exposure by choosing "light" tuna instead of white albacore because it tends to contain lower amounts of mercury. If your kids like only albacore, the FDA advises giving them no more than one serving per week. And don't rely solely on canned tuna for their fish servings. Serve other kinds of lower-mercury fish such as salmon and tilapia too.

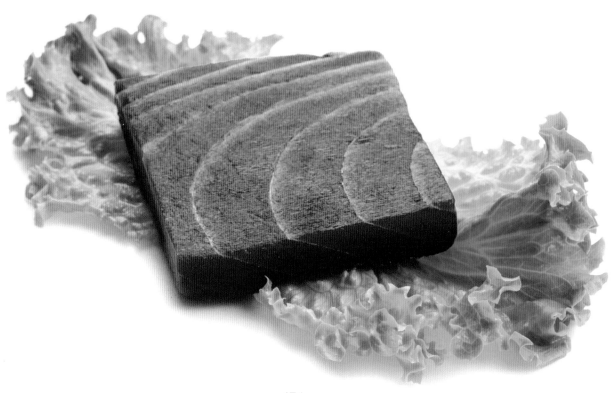

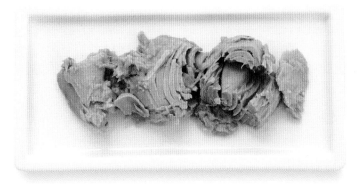

WHAT'S A SERVING OF FISH FOR KIDS?

- Ages 2–3: 1 ounce (28 g)
- Ages 4–7: 2 ounces (55 g)
- Ages 8–10: 3 ounces (85 g)
- Ages 11 and up: 4 ounces (115 g)

Source: FDA

Q: Should I Be Worried about Mercury in Fish?

Most fish contain some amount of methylmercury, which can be toxic to the brain in large amounts. Really big fish tend to pack the most mercury because they live a long time and gobble up lots of smaller fish. So the FDA advises against eating these fish: tilefish from the Gulf of Mexico, shark, swordfish, orange roughy, marlin, bigeye tuna, and king mackerel. But other varieties have smaller amounts and are safe even for very young kids. Some fish and seafood with the lowest amounts include:

- Salmon (Atlantic, chinook, coho, pink, sockeye)
- Tilapia
- Pollock (Atlantic and walleye)
- Flounder
- Haddock
- Catfish
- Clams
- Oysters
- Shrimp
- Scallops (bay and sea)

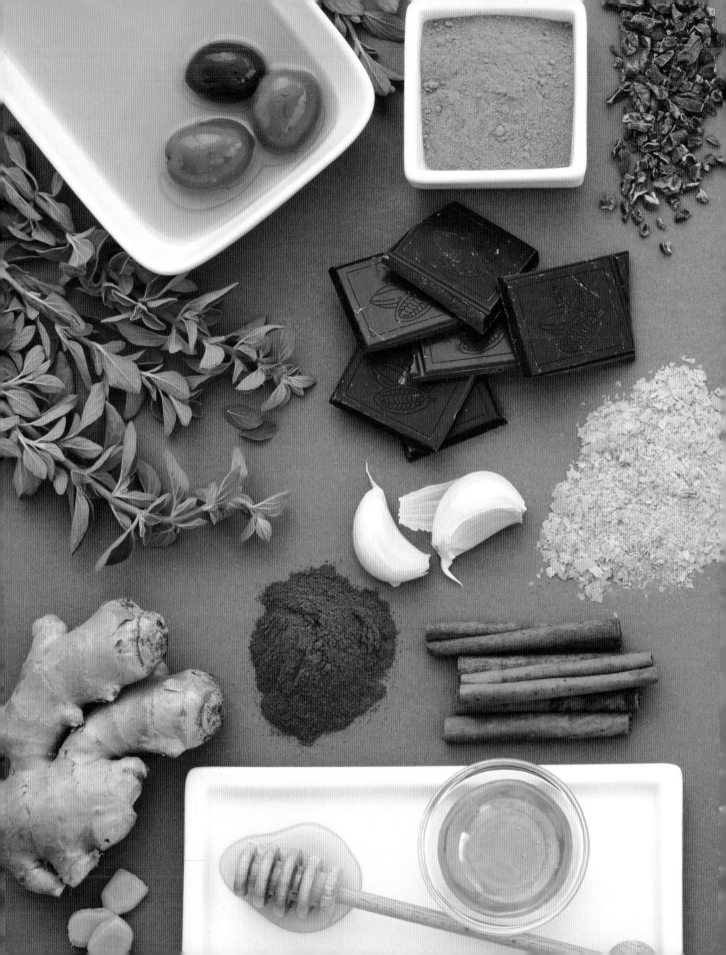

5

Spices & Seasonings

MANY BABIES (INCLUDING MINE) STARTED OUT

on spoonfuls of rice cereal. Plain, safe, hypoallergenic—and totally bland and boring. In hindsight, I wish I'd served my two boys more flavorful foods in those first months of starting solids so they would have developed a palate for spices and seasonings from an early age. That's handy, not only because it makes family meals a lot easier (no need to leave out the chili pepper or skip the smoky paprika) but also because so many of the herbs and spices added to food are naturally infused with health-protective powers. Your spice cabinet may not provide your child with fiber, vitamin C, or calcium, because the quantities we add to foods are too small to give us significant amounts. But it is brimming with compounds that scientists believe have healing and disease-fighting capabilities. And besides, seasonings simply make meals more interesting—and can make healthy foods taste even better.

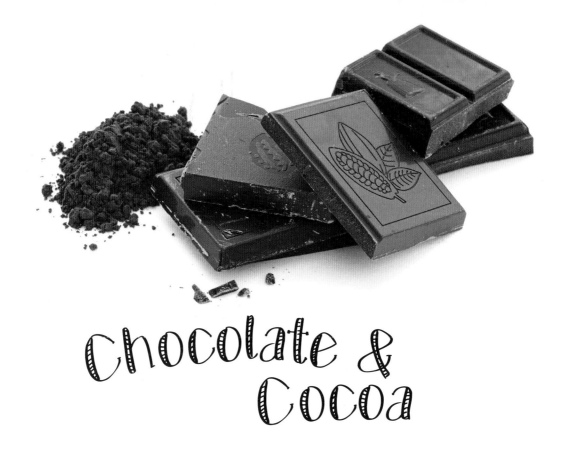

Chocolate & Cocoa

I can't give you the green light to sprinkle M&Ms on everything. But I can assure you that chocolate and cocoa *can* have a place in a healthy diet (release the confetti!). Chocolate and cocoa powder both come from cocoa beans, which are **rich in magnesium** and contain iron, calcium, and potassium. And though chocolate is rich in fat thanks to cocoa butter, it contains a kind of saturated fat called stearic acid that doesn't raise blood cholesterol levels in the same way other kinds might.

Like all plants, cocoa beans also possess unique health-boosting compounds such as flavanols that work as antioxidants and may have some **protective effects on heart health**, including improving blood flow. But not all chocolate is necessarily rich in flavanols. Dark chocolate is more likely to pack them because it contains more cacao (cocoa bean) and less sugar. In fact, experts recommend choosing chocolate with at least 70 percent cacao to get more of the health benefits. Semisweet chocolate will have fewer protective compounds, followed by milk chocolate. White chocolate will have none because it doesn't contain any cocoa bean solids and isn't actually "chocolate" at all, just cocoa butter, sugar, and flavorings. Cocoa powder labeled "natural" also packs flavanols, but "Dutch processed" or "alkalized" cocoa (which is more commonly used) has far fewer. Yet cocoa powder is still a great way to impart a rich chocolate flavor without any added sugar—and has two grams of fiber and a bit of iron per tablespoon (5 g) to boot!

Chocolate Breakfast Shake

A thick, frosty shake for breakfast? Sure thing, when it is made with real cocoa and cinnamon, includes nourishing ingredients that provide protein and fiber for fullness, and is sweetened without any added sugar.

1 cup (235 ml) milk (dairy or nondairy)
1 frozen banana, broken in half
2 teaspoons unsweetened cocoa powder
1/8 teaspoon ground cinnamon
2 pitted dates, soaked overnight*
3 tablespoons (30 g) oats

Place the milk, banana, cocoa powder, cinnamon, dates, and oats in a blender in the order listed. Blend until smooth. Serve immediately.

*Soak your dates overnight so they'll blend more easily. Place them in a small dish of milk, cover, and refrigerate overnight or for at least 8 hours. You can also just soak them for a few minutes in hot water if you didn't have time to plan ahead.

Yield: 1 serving

Q: Is Caffeine Safe for Kids?

A little bit is okay—but a lot definitely isn't. Caffeine can be hard on kids' smaller systems, increasing blood pressure, wrecking sleep, and even causing dependency and withdrawal symptoms such as headaches. There aren't official U.S. recommendations for kids and caffeine, but Health Canada suggests no more than 45 mg a day for kids ages four to six, 62.5 mg for kids ages seven to nine, and 85 mg for kids ten to twelve. A typical soda contains between 30 and 60 mg for a regular can (the ubiquitous 20-ounce bottles obviously have a lot more). Frozen coffee shop drinks pack about 100. Just be sure your child steers clear of energy drinks, which the American Academy of Pediatrics advises against for all kids.

Good to Know

If you've come across a recipe that calls for "cacao nibs" or seen bags of them at the natural foods store, here's the scoop: Cacao nibs are dried, roasted, and crushed up cocoa beans. Though they can be used in place of chocolate chips, they don't contain any added sugar—so they have a deep, intense flavor, but they're not sweet.

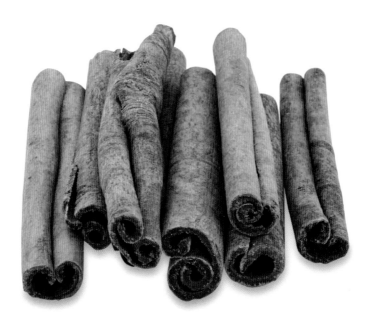

Cinnamon

The simple spice you sprinkle on your child's toast in the morning has been used for centuries as both a flavoring agent and a home remedy. Though most of the research on cinnamon has been done in animals or test tubes (and not people), there's evidence that cinnamon might help lower cholesterol, regulate blood sugar, and reduce inflammation. In research from Touro College in New York City, the spice was even shown to deactivate viruses by destroying their outer coating—so it might even offer **defense against the kinds of viruses that cause colds and flu**.

What we know for sure: Cinnamon is an affordable spice that adds lots of flavor to food and even a hint of sweetness without using sugar. Sprinkle it on your child's oatmeal or yogurt, or whirl it into smoothies, for a sugar-free kick.

Good to Know

Read labels carefully on foods marketed as "reduced sugar." Instead of just cutting back on added sugars, some manufactures also include artificial sweeteners such as sucralose, aspartame, and acesulfame potassium to make up the differences. If you want to avoid faux sweeteners, look out for those ingredients in products such as reduced-sugar juice, ketchup, and canned fruit.

"TRY IT" TIP

Sprinkle apple slices with cinnamon before packing them in your child's lunch box. Not only will the cinnamon give the apples a flavor kick, but it will also disguise any unappealing browning that may occur.

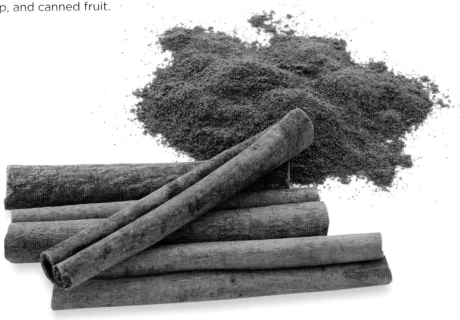

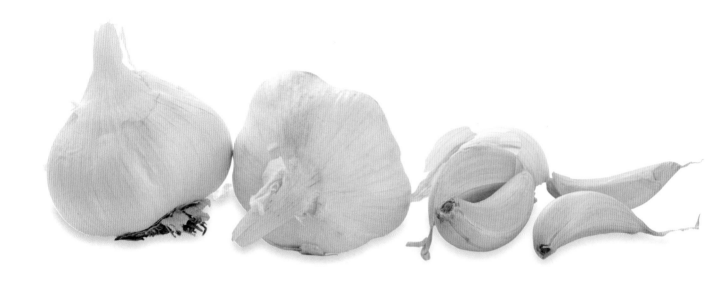

Garlic

The health benefits of garlic don't come from vitamins and minerals (the amounts are too tiny to be meaningful) but from the natural plant chemicals it contains. Garlic has been used for thousands of years to treat a wide number of ailments, and research shows it likely does have some medicinal powers. For instance, one of the major bioactive components of garlic, called allicin, has been shown to have **antimicrobial effects against bacteria, fungi, and viruses**. Some population studies also show an association between eating garlic and lower rates of some cancers.

You'll get the most benefit from fresh garlic—even more if you mince or crush it because that increases the surface area (it also means more flavor). Bonus points if you can chop your garlic in advance because it takes about 15 minutes for the allicin to develop after it's been cut.

Easy Peanut Sauce

In our house, we drizzle this simple sauce on rice and veggie bowls. It's a sweet way to encourage kids to eat their veggies.

¼ cup (16 g) natural peanut butter
3 tablespoons (60 g) real maple syrup
3 tablespoons (45 ml) reduced-sodium soy sauce
1 teaspoon rice vinegar
1 teaspoon sesame oil
1 clove garlic, minced or pressed
1 tablespoon (15 ml) water (optional)

In a small bowl, whisk together the peanut butter, maple syrup, soy sauce, vinegar, oil, and garlic until smooth. If the sauce is too thick, drizzle in water slowly, 1 teaspoon at a time, while whisking, until you get the texture you like.

Yield: About ⅔ cup (160 ml)

 "TRY IT" TIP

If your child's not a fan of the strong flavor of garlic, try roasting it to bring out the natural sweetness. Remove the loose outer layers from a head of garlic (keeping the skins on), cut off the tops to expose the cloves, drizzle with olive oil, and wrap the whole thing in foil. Place the bundle on a baking sheet and roast at 400°F (200°C) for about 30 minutes. It's done when the cloves are soft and easily pierced with a fork. Use the roasted garlic in your recipes or spread it on bread along with butter.

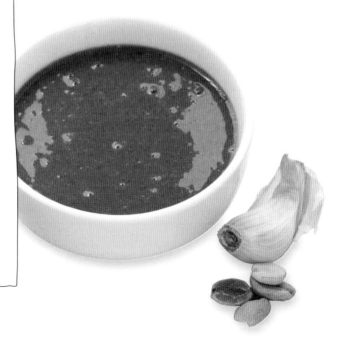

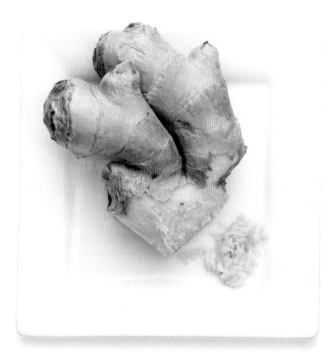

Ginger

Ginger is thought of as a root but is technically an herb. And like many other herbs, it's been used for thousands of years as a natural remedy for everything from colds and coughs to nausea.

There are more than 100 components of ginger that have been identified, but gingerols—which give ginger its strong, spicy smell—are the main bioactive component. Gingerols have been studied for their potential to alleviate pain, act as an anti-inflammatory, lower cholesterol, and even suppress the growth of cancer cells. But ginger is best known as a home remedy for nausea, including motion sickness and morning sickness. Some research shows it's as effective at **combating queasiness** as over-the-counter meds, while other research refutes this. But since ginger doesn't typically have any adverse effects, it's worth a shot! Keep in mind that most ginger ale has little to no actual ginger in it. You can brew your own ginger tea by steeping one-half to one teaspoon of grated ginger in a cup of hot water for several minutes, straining it out, and then adding a touch of honey for sweetness.

After buying ginger, store it at room temperature. The easiest way to remove the outer skin is to peel it off using a paring knife or the back of a spoon. To use ginger, blend a small knob of it into smoothies for a spicy kick. You can also mince or grate some into stir-fries.

Honey

I cringe when I see recipes billed as "healthy" just because they're made with honey instead of white sugar. Using honey in place of white sugar doesn't automatically make brownies, fudge, or doughnuts healthy. Honey earns a spot in this book because it does boast some nutrients and unique benefits compared to other forms of added sugar—but that's not license to pour it on with reckless abandon. It is still an added sugar and should be used in small amounts, like other sweeteners. Since honey is sweeter than table sugar, though, you may be able to use less.

According to research, honey contains more than 180 different substances, and these vary depending on the season, climate, and flowers the bees used to extract nectar. Some of these substances may have the **power to work as antioxidants and antimicrobials**.

Buy raw honey if it's affordable to you, but don't worry if you can't. Though some of the antioxidant power is reduced when honey is processed, research shows the antioxidants are still available to the body.

Consider turning to honey the next time your child has a cough and can't sleep. In a study published in *Pediatrics*, children one to five years of age who had upper respiratory infections were given either honey or a placebo at bedtime. Parents whose children got honey reported that their kids **coughed less frequently and severely**. They also slept better (and just as importantly, so did the parents!). Just remember to never give honey to a child younger than one. Honey may contain spores that can cause botulism in a baby's still-developing digestive tract.

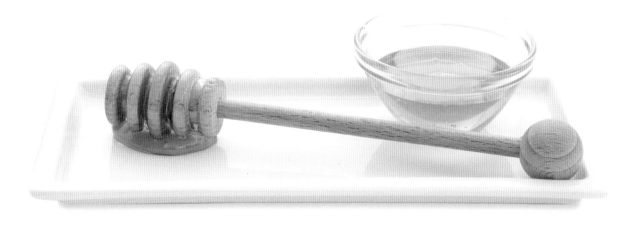

Nutritional Yeast

It's a fact: Nutritional yeast sort of looks like fish food. Once you get past that, you and your kids will probably love this savory flavoring that tastes cheesy but is totally vegan. Affectionately called "nooch" by its tribe of devotees, nutritional yeast is a deactivated form of yeast, so it's different from the yeast used to make bread.

For such silly-sounding stuff, it's got some decent nutritional cred. One tablespoon (8 g) has about two grams of protein and one gram of fiber. Nutritional yeast is also fortified with B vitamins. That makes it **a friend to vegetarians and vegans**, who are often missing out on B_{12}, which is found in animal foods. Nutritional yeast is also typically **gluten free**. Look for nutritional yeast in a powder or flake form in the natural foods section of your grocery store, natural foods market, health food store, and online. My kids clamor for it sprinkled over home-popped popcorn. You can also shake it onto roasted veggies, into scrambled eggs, and over potatoes. Or use it to create a dairy-free sauce for mac and cheese or vegetables.

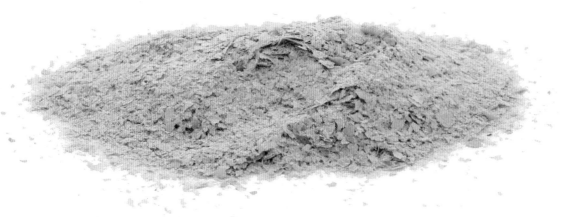

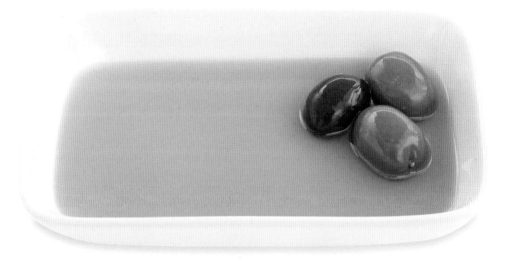

Olive Oil

Like the fruit they come from, olive oil is **rich in heart-healthy monounsaturated fat**. According to the FDA, two tablespoons (30 ml) a day can reduce the risk of heart disease when it replaces sources of saturated fat such as butter and lard. Olive oil is also packed with **protective compounds such as polyphenols**. Along with fruits, vegetables, nuts, seeds, fish, seafood, whole grains, and healthy fats such as avocados, olive oil is a key part of the Mediterranean Diet, which has been shown to help protect against a host of diseases and conditions including heart disease, diabetes, and some cancers.

Extra-virgin olive oil, made from the first pressing of the olives, is considered the healthiest variety of olive oil because it packs more polyphenols. It's best reserved for dressings or drizzling on at the end of cooking. Regular olive oil can be used for cooking but likely contains fewer disease-fighting compounds once heated. "Light" olive oil simply means it's lighter in flavor, not that it's lower in calories or fat. Whichever you choose, keep the bottle in a dark spot such as the pantry to protect it from quality-degrading light and buy only an amount you can use within one to two months.

Good to Know

There are claims that some oils labeled "olive oil" actually aren't. To be sure you're getting the real deal, look on the bottle for a harvest date and country of origin (preferably the specific estate where it comes from).

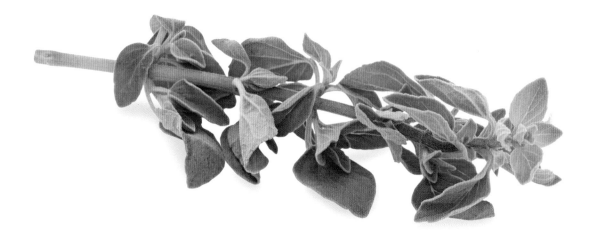

Oregano

This strong-flavored herb is a staple of Italian cooking and has some surprisingly potent benefits: Research published in the *Journal of Agricultural and Food Chemistry* found that the herb has a high **antioxidant activity,** just as fruits and vegetables such as apples, oranges, and even blueberries do. It may also have some **natural antibacterial powers.** Oregano oil damaged illness-causing bacteria such as E. coli when scientists put them together in test tubes. Even a small amount of the herb sprinkled onto food provides some nutrients: One teaspoon of dried oregano contains a little bit of **calcium, iron, and vitamin K** (a vitamin that helps with proper blood clotting).

A member of the mint family, oregano is a no-brainer for pasta, pizza, and homemade Italian salad dressing. But you can also add it to tomato soup, chili, and chicken dishes. If you're buying fresh oregano, get only as much as you can use quickly. Stored in a plastic bag in the refrigerator, it will keep for about three days. Dried oregano obviously has a much longer shelf life: It will last up to three years in a cool, dry spot (you'll know it's still good to use if it has retained its color and has a pungent aroma when you sniff it). If your recipe calls for fresh oregano but you only have dried, use one-third of the amount. For example, if your recipe specifies one tablespoon fresh oregano, swap in one teaspoon of dried oregano.

Homemade Pizza Sauce

Keep a jar of this zesty sauce in the fridge for homemade pizza night or to spoon onto bagel halves or whole wheat pita, top with cheese, and place under the broiler for a quick after-school snack. If your kids don't like any chunks of tomato in their sauces, whirl the crushed tomatoes in the blender until smooth before using.

2 teaspoons olive oil
1 medium clove garlic, minced or pressed
1 can (15 ounces [429 g]) crushed tomatoes
2 tablespoons (32 g) tomato paste
1 tablespoon (3 g) dried oregano
1/2 teaspoon dried onion powder
1/2 teaspoon salt
1/4 teaspoon ground pepper
Big pinch of white sugar (optional)

In a medium saucepan, heat the olive oil over medium heat. Add the garlic, cooking and stirring for 30 seconds. Add the tomatoes, tomato paste, oregano, onion powder, salt, pepper, and sugar (if using) and stir to combine. Reduce the heat to low and simmer the sauce for 30 minutes, stirring occasionally.

Yield: 1 1/2 cups (355 ml)

Good to Know

To keep fresh basil, parsley, or cilantro looking and tasting fresh, trim the stems and place them in a glass or jar of water, like you would with cut flowers. Loosely cover it with a plastic bag and keep refrigerated.

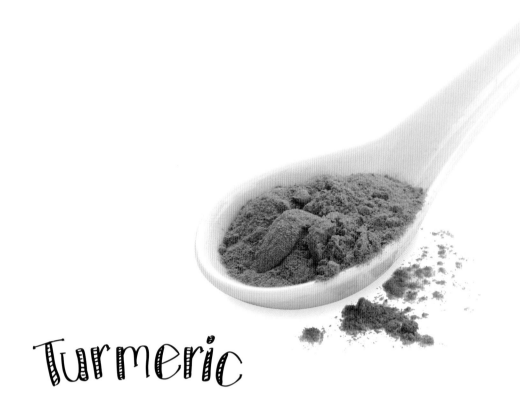

Turmeric

Even if you don't keep this spice in your kitchen cabinet, chances are you've already had it. Turmeric is what gives Indian curry dishes their vivid yellow color, and it's widely used by food manufacturers as a natural food color in place of synthetic food dyes such as Yellow #5. Though it's recently become trendy here in the United States, it's been used for thousands of years as both a spice and a natural remedy in Eastern medicine.

The active compound in turmeric is curcumin, which research has found may act as a **natural antioxidant** and **anti-inflammatory**. Scientists are studying whether curcumin may help reduce the risk for conditions such as heart disease and some cancer and offer relief from ailments including indigestion, arthritis, and even depression. Though the research has largely been done with turmeric extract—a dose you'd find in a supplement, much more than you'd get from a shake or two of the spice—there's no doubt that turmeric adds a rich and vibrant color to dishes and may have some health benefits to boot. Some research has found that you'll absorb curcumin even better from turmeric when you consume black pepper along with it.

Q: Should I Avoid Synthetic Food Dyes?

I think it makes sense to avoid foods and drinks with synthetic dyes when you can—and luckily there are plenty of alternative products formulated with natural colors from plants (like turmeric!). Though synthetic food dyes have been in the food supply for many decades, questions and controversy have swirled around them. Most recently, a large analysis of studies from Oregon Health and Science University in Portland found an association between the dyes and symptoms of inattention among children. The FDA has also acknowledged that some food additives may affect vulnerable children. My personal policy: I'm not bothered by an occasional dyed cupcake at a party, but I don't typically stock any dyed foods or drinks at home.

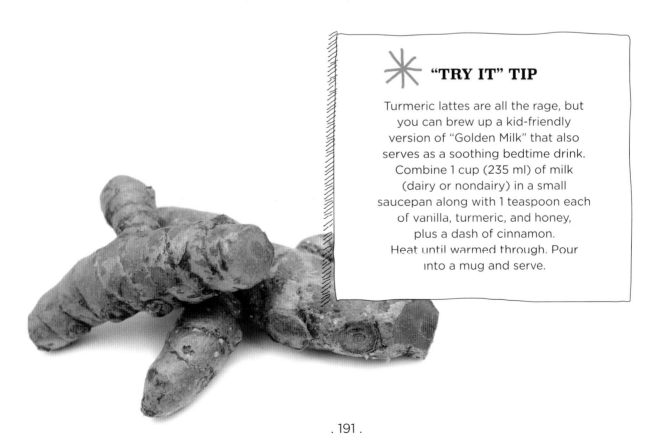

✳ "TRY IT" TIP

Turmeric lattes are all the rage, but you can brew up a kid-friendly version of "Golden Milk" that also serves as a soothing bedtime drink. Combine 1 cup (235 ml) of milk (dairy or nondairy) in a small saucepan along with 1 teaspoon each of vanilla, turmeric, and honey, plus a dash of cinnamon. Heat until warmed through. Pour into a mug and serve.

Top 10 Lists

10 Foods to Ease Constipation

It's a common problem among kids and a source of belly pain, gas, and bloating. To help ease it naturally, you'll want to give your child plenty of foods rich in fiber, which makes stools soft, bulky, and easier to pass. If your child isn't used to eating fiber-rich foods, add them slowly to avoid GI problems. Be sure your child is drinking plenty of fluids too, which are key for staying regular.

1. Raspberries

2. Oatmeal

3. Whole wheat pasta

4. Potatoes (with the skin)

5. Flaxseed

6. Pears

7. Refried beans

8. Popcorn

9. Lentils

10. Apples (with the skin)

10 Foods for Extra Iron

Growing kids need iron, a mineral that helps the body deliver oxygen to cells. Iron is critical during the first few years of life, and needs a jump during adolescence for girls. There are two kinds of iron: Heme iron is found in animal foods and is well absorbed by the body. Nonheme is the kind in plant foods and isn't soaked up by the body—but you can boost absorption by pairing it with another food rich in vitamin C, such as berries, sweet peppers, spinach, or potatoes.

1. Fortified breakfast cereal

2. Lentils

3. Tofu

4. Beans

5. Beef

6. Chickpeas

7. Chicken

8. Pork

9. Spinach

10. Raisins

10 Foods for Boosting Immunity

There are many nutrients and compounds involved in keeping the immune system healthy and bugs at bay, and these foods are brimming with them.

1. Yogurt

2. Sweet potatoes

3. Beef

4. Strawberries

5. Ginger

6. Mushrooms

7. Grapefruit

8. Oranges

9. Garlic

10. Beans

10 Foods for Post-Game Refueling

The smartest post-game meal or snack combines protein to help repair and rebuild muscles plus carbohydrates to restock depleted energy stores.

1. Yogurt with fresh or frozen berries

2. Peanut butter and jelly spread on a whole wheat tortilla and rolled up

3. Cheese stick or slices with whole grain crackers

4. Popcorn with a glass of chocolate milk

5. Deli meat sandwich on whole wheat bread

6. Apple slices with almond butter or sunflower butter

7. Cottage cheese and sliced peaches

8. Hummus or bean dip and pita

9. Small bowl of cereal with milk

10. Trail mix made with nuts, dried fruit, and whole grain cereal pieces

10 Foods for Brain Building

These foods don't guarantee early admission to an Ivy League school, but they all contain nutrients and substances that have been linked to brain development and better learning and memory—or that can help children stay full and focused so it's easier to learn.

1. Blueberries and wild blueberries

2. Oats

3. Eggs

4. Tuna

5. Salmon

6. Beef

7. Beans

8. Lentils

9. Edamame

10. Flaxseed

10 Foods that Aren't as Healthy as They Seem

Watch out for packaged foods hyped up to be healthy. Always read the ingredient list and Nutrition Facts panel to see what's really inside.

1. Fruit juice

2. Granola

3. Gummy fruit snacks

4. Veggie chips

5. Energy bars

6. "Wheat" bread

7. "Multigrain" bread

8. Diet soda

9. Protein bars and powder

10. Frozen yogurt

10 Foods for Road Trips

Fill a bag with these healthy shelf-stable foods for munching on during long car trips.

1. Popcorn

2. Fresh fruit such as apples, clementines, and bananas

3. Beef jerky

4. Nuts

5. Dried fruit and freeze-dried fruit

6. Unsweetened applesauce cups

7. Whole grain crackers

8. Shelf-stable boxes of milk and chocolate milk

9. Homemade trail mix

10. Container of whole grain cereal

10 Foods for Bedtime

The best bedtime snacks are light, easy to digest, and rich in relaxing carbohydrates.

1. Whole grain crackers

2. Glass of milk warmed with a drop or two of vanilla extract

3. Small bowl of yogurt with fruit

4. Half of a whole grain bagel spread with nut butter

5. Cup of cottage cheese with berries

6. Small bowl of cereal with milk

7. Half of a nut butter sandwich

8. Small bowl of popcorn

9. Small whole grain pita spread with hummus

10. Banana

Resources

For more advice, here are some of my favorite books about feeding kids:

It's Not about the Broccoli by Dina Rose

Fearless Feeding by Jill Castle and Maryann Jacobsen

Getting to Yum by Karen Le Billon

Child of Mine by Ellyn Satter

Raising a Healthy, Happy Eater by Nimali Fernando and Melanie Potock

The Picky Eater Project by Natalie Digate Muth and Sally Sampson

Helping Your Child with Extreme Picky Eating by Katja Rowell and Jenny McGlothlin

Born to Eat by Leslie Schilling and Wendy Jo Peterson

Baby-Led Feeding by Jenna Helwig

Acknowledgments

A sincere note of thanks to the following people:

Katherine Petro for your time and hard work.

Carolyn Williams for your wordsmith talent and RD input.

Katie Morford for your friendship, wisdom, and pep talks.

My kid recipe testers, Ezra Phillips, Rachel Husenits, and Ella Amodei, and to their moms, Courtney, Melissa, and Michelle, for making it all happen (and probably cleaning up afterward).

My editor, Amanda Waddell, and the team at Fair Winds Press for making this experience such a pleasure.

My agent, Carole Bidnick, for your ongoing support.

Jesseca Salky for your expertise and advice.

My parents, Ron and Lucille, for bragging about me around town.

My kids, Henry and Sam, for tolerating the endless requests to "Please take a bite of this; I'm testing it for the book" and keeping me humble by not always liking what I make for dinner.

My husband, Joel, for too many things to list here, but especially for convincing me ten years ago that I should start something called a blog and for doing all the dishes.

About the Author

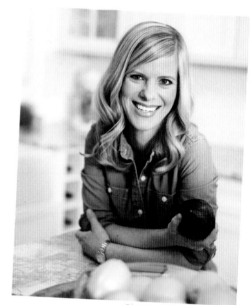

Photo by Lauryn Byrdy

SALLY KUZEMCHAK, M.S., R.D., is a registered dietitian, author, and educator. She blogs at RealMomNutrition.com, a "no-judgments zone" about feeding a family that was voted Best Blog for Parents by *Health* magazine in 2015 and named in the Best of the Web Awards by *Parents* magazine in 2016. In 2014, she collaborated with *Cooking Light* on *Dinnertime Survival Guide,* a cookbook for busy families. An award-winning reporter and writer, Sally has been published in nearly 20 magazines including *Prevention, Family Circle, Eating Well, Fitness,* and *Shape* and currently serves as a contributing editor for *Parents* magazine. Sally received her master's degree in dietetics from The Ohio State University and has served as adjunct faculty at Otterbein University and Ohio University Lancaster. She lives in Columbus, Ohio, with her husband and two young boys, one of whom likes meat and starch, and one of whom likes veggies, so at least together, they eat a balanced meal.

Index

A

Actinidin, 92
Almond milk, 157, 165
Almonds, 156–157
Alpha-linolenic acid (ALA), 160, 163
Ancient grains, 124
Anthocyanins, 28, 30, 50, 52, 76, 78, 82, 90, 98, 136
Antibacterial powers, 188. *See also* Bacteria in the gut; Prebiotics; Probiotics
Anticancer powers. *See* Cancer-fighting foods
Anti-inflammatories, 80, 82, 104, 164, 190
Antioxidants/antioxidant power, 18, 20, 22, 30, 38, 50, 52, 56, 59, 68–69, 74–75, 76, 78, 79, 80, 82, 86, 93, 96, 110, 125, 132, 136, 150, 155, 178, 185, 188, 190. *See also* Anthocyanins; Beta-carotene; Lycopene; Polyphenols
Appetites, 117
Apples, 68–69, 133, 181, 192, 195
Applesauce, 69, 153, 198
Apricots, 70–71
Arsenic, in rice, 119
Asparagus, 18–19
Avocados, 72–73

B

Baba ghanoush, 41
Babies
    beef for, 137
    fish eaten by, 171
    juice for, 69
    peanut protein and, 158
    yogurt and, 147
Baby carrots, 31
Bacteria in the gut, 45, 52, 68, 146. *See also* Prebiotics; Probiotics
Bananas, 74–75, 199
Barley, 116–117
Beans, 136, 194, 196
Bedtime, 10 foods for, 199

Beef, 137, 194, 196
Beef jerky, 198
Beets, 20–21
Beta-carotene, 20, 26, 30, 54, 61, 62, 70, 88, 95
Beta-cryptoxanthin, 26
Beta-glucan, 116, 126
Betalains, 20
Blackberries, 76–77
Blueberries
    about, 78
    adding to pancakes or muffins, 79
    Berry and Beet Smoothie, 21
    Blueberry Banana "Ice Cream," 75
    for brain building, 196
    wild, 79
Blueberry Banana "Ice Cream," 75
Brain building foods, 78, 137, 150, 170, 196
BRAT diet, 74
Broccoli, 22
Broccolini, 21
Bromelain, 104
Brown eggs, 151
Brown rice, 118
Brussels sprouts, 24–25
Buddha bowls, 118
Bulgur, 120
Butter, 61
Butternut squash, 26–27
B vitamins, 36, 86, 116, 118, 186. *See also* Folate

C

Cabbage, 28–29
Cacao nibs, 179
Caesar salad, 56
Caffeine, 179
Calcium, 20, 22, 42, 44, 46, 56, 57, 82, 84, 86, 98, 136, 138, 140, 141, 142, 144, 145, 146, 156, 188
Cancer-fighting foods, 19, 20, 22, 24, 26, 28, 32, 46, 50, 54, 59, 62, 68, 82, 90, 93, 94, 110, 112, 163, 168, 184
Canned vegetables, 43

Cantaloupe, 80–81
Carbohydrates, 127
Carrots, 30–31
Cauliflower, 32–33
Cavities, 133
Celery, 34–35
Celiac disease, 116, 122, 123, 128
Cereal, 133, 193, 195, 198
Cherries, 82–83
Chia seeds, 162
Chickpeas, 138–139, 169, 194
Chinese gooseberry, 92
Chips
    Cheesy Brussels Sprouts Chips, 25
    Crunchy Kale Chips, 47
    veggie chips, 41
Cholesterol
    coconut and, 84
    eggs and, 150
Cholesterol-lowering foods, 20, 72, 96,
    116, 126, 136, 138, 155, 156, 158, 166,
    168, 172, 180, 184
Cinnamon, 180
Clementines, 98
Cocoa powder, 178
Coconut, 84–85
Coconut milk, 84
Coconut oil, 85
Coconut sugar, 85
Constipation, 102, 107, 126, 156, 167, 192
"Converted" rice, 119
Corn, 36–37
Cottage cheese, 140, 141, 195, 199
Couscous, 122
Crackers, whole grain, 198, 199
Cucumbers, 38–39
Curcumin, 190
Curly kale, 46, 47

D
Dairy-free milks, 165
Dark chocolate, 178
Dates, 86
Dehydrated veggies, 41
Diarrhea, 74
Diet soda, 197
Docosahexaenoic acid (DHA), 170
Dried apricots, 70
Dried fruit, 83, 198

"Dried" plums, 107
"Dutch processed" cocoa powder, 178

E
Easy Peanut Sauce, 118, 183
Eating habits, ten healthy eating rules, 15
Edamame, 148, 196
Eggplant, 40–41
Eggs, 150–151, 163, 196
Eicosapentaenoic acid (EPA), 170
Energy bars, 197
Ethylene, 102, 111
Extra-virgin olive oil, 187

F
Family, eating as a, 15
Farmed salmon, 170–171
Farro, 124
Fiber, 102, 108, 118, 120, 122, 124, 125, 132,
    136, 138, 148, 152, 162, 163
Fish, 170–171, 174–175
Flavanols, 178
Flavored milk, 145
Flaxseed, 163, 192, 196
Folate, 18, 19, 20, 22, 26, 32, 34, 50, 64,
    98, 110, 136, 152
Food labels. *See* Labels
Fortified breakfast cereal, 193
Fortified kefir, 142
Fortified milk, 144
Fortified orange juice, 98
Fortified soy milk, 145
Freeze-dried fruit, 198
French fries, 53
Frozen bananas, 75
Frozen berries, 77, 78
Frozen grapes, 91
Frozen vegetables, 43, 57
Frozen yogurt, 197
Fructans, 51
Fruit juice, 98, 197
Fruit kebabs, 81
Fruit snacks, 71, 197
Fruits, recommended daily intake, 67.
    See also specific names of fruits
Full-fat milk, 144

G

Gamma-linolenic acid (GLA), 164
Garlic, 182, 194
Ginger, 184, 194
Ginger tea, 184
Glucosinolates, 22
Glutathione, 19
Gluten, 116, 122, 123
Gluten-free foods, 36, 125, 126, 128, 132, 152, 186
Grains, recommended daily intake, 115. *See also* specific types of grains
Granola, 197
Grapefruit, 88–89, 194
Grapefruit juice, 88
Grapes, 90–91
Greek yogurt, 146–147
Green beans, 42–43
Green peas, 44
Guacamole, 73
Gummy fruit snacks, 71, 197

H

Hemp seeds, 164
Honey, 185
Honeydew, 80–81
Hummus, 195, 199
Hunger, 117

I

Ice pops, 104–105
Immunity, 10 foods for boosting, 194
Insoluble fiber, 36, 102, 107, 126, 136
Instant oats, 126
"Instant" rice, 119
Inulin, 45
Iron, 18, 46, 54, 57, 58, 70, 86, 88, 91, 107, 118, 120, 122, 124, 125, 133, 136, 137, 138, 148, 149, 155, 160, 162, 164, 166, 170, 174, 178, 188, 193
Irritable bowel syndrome, 51
Israeli couscous, 122

J

Jicama, 34
Juice
  grapefruit, 88
  limiting, 69
  not as healthy as it seems, 197
  "not from concentrate" label, 99
  orange, 98, 99
  pomegranate, 108
"Just one bite rule," 47

K

Kale, 36–37
Kebabs, fruit, 81
Kefir, 142–143
Ketchup, 63
Kiwifruit, 92
Kohlrabi, 48

L

Labels
  "hormone free," 151
  juice, 99
  "live and active cultures," 146
  "made with whole grain" on, 121
  olive oils, 187
  peanut/nut free and, 166, 167
  "reduced sugar," 181
  sugar(s) and, 87, 103, 181
  tahini, 168
  "whole wheat" on, 130
Lacinato kale, 46
Lactose intolerance, 141
Lemon juice, 102
Lemons, 93
Lentils, 152–154, 192, 193, 196
Lettuce, romaine, 56
"Light" olive oil, 187
Lignans, 54, 168
Limes, 93
Limonene, 93
Lutein, 30, 56, 57, 150, 155
Lycopene, 30, 43, 59, 62, 88, 94, 112

M

Magnesium, 13, 30, 36, 40, 45, 56, 64, 84, 100, 102, 118, 120, 125, 136, 144, 148, 156, 160, 164, 166, 168, 178
Malted beverages, 116
Malt vinegar, 116
Mandarins, 98
Manganese, 78, 104
Mango, 95
Meals, serving just one, 15, 29
Medications, grapefruit and, 89

Mediterranean Diet, 96
Medjool dates, 86
Mercury, 174, 175
Milk, 144–145, 199. *See also* Dairy-free milks
Milk chocolate, 178
Millet, 125
Monounsaturated fat, 72, 96, 158, 166, 187
"Multigrain" bread, 197
Multivitamins, 51
Mushrooms, 49, 137, 194

N

Nausea, ginger for, 184
Navel oranges, 98
New foods, encouraging children to try, 13–14
Niacin, 86, 156, 174
Nuggets, cauliflower, 33
Nut butters, 157, 199
Nutritional yeast, 186

O

Oatmeal, 192
Oats, 126–127, 196
Olive oil, 187
Olives, 96–97
Omega-3 fats, 54, 149, 160, 162, 163, 164, 170–171, 174
Onions, 50–51
Orange juice, 98, 99
Oranges, 98–99, 194
Oregano, 188
Organic eggs, 150
Organic vegetables, 60
Oxalic acid, 57

P

Paleo diet, 121
Pancakes, oatmeal, 127
Pancakes, Pumpkin Chocolate Chip, 55
Papain, 94
Papaya, 94
Parboiled rice, 119
Pasta, 131
Peaches, 100–101
Peanut butter
  Easy Peanut Sauce, 183
  Homemade Peanut Butter, 159

as post-game meal/snack, 195
  Red Lentil Snack Cookies, 153
  served as a dip with veggies, 159
  weight status and, 158
Peanut protein, 158
Peanuts, 158–159
Pearl couscous, 122
Pearled barley, 116
Pears, 102–103, 192
Pectin, 68, 74, 102
Pepitas, 54
Peppers, 58–59
Phytosterols, 72, 155, 166, 168
Pickled beets, 20
Picky eating, 12, 14, 39. *See also* "Try it" tips
Pineapple, 104–105
Pistachios, 155
Plant protein, 136
Plums, 106
Polyphenols, 30, 90, 108, 124, 187
Pomegranate juice, 108
Pomegranates, 108–109
Popcorn, 37, 195, 198, 199
Pork, 194
Post-game foods, 195
Potassium, 20, 26, 32, 36, 38, 42, 46, 48, 52, 53, 54, 62, 64, 68, 70, 72, 74, 82, 84, 86, 88, 91, 92, 94, 95, 98, 100, 108, 137, 144, 148, 155, 166, 178
Potatoes, 52–53, 192
Prebiotics, 45, 51, 102, 143, 156
Probiotics, 29, 39, 51, 142, 143
Protein
  foods providing, 22, 24, 44, 54, 57, 120, 122, 124, 125, 128, 130, 135–176, 186, 195
  recommended daily amount, 135
Protein bars, 197
Protein powder, 154, 197
Prunes, 107
Pumpkin, 54–55

Q

Quercetin, 50, 82
Quick oats, 126
Quinoa, 128–129

R

Raisins, 91, 194
Raspberries, 76–77, 147, 192
Raw honey, 185
Raw milk, 145
Recipes
  Baked Quinoa Bites, 129
  Berry and Beet Smoothie, 21
  Better-for-You Orange Julius, 99
  Blueberry Banana "Ice Cream," 75
  Broiled Grapefruit, 89
  Brown Bag Popcorn, 37
  cauliflower nuggets, 33
  Cheesy Brussels Sprouts Chips, 25
  Chocolate Breakfast Shake, 179
  Easy Peanut Sauce, 183
  Easy Peasy Hummus, 169
  Game-Changing Roasted Broccoli, 23
  Homemade Peanut Butter, 159
  Homemade Pizza Sauce, 189
  Homemade Tortillas, 131
  Make-Ahead Instant Oatmeal Pancakes, 127
  Melted Berry Sauce, 111
  Nut-Free Snack Balls, 167
  Pumpkin Chocolate Chip Pancakes, 55
  Red Lentil Snack Cookies, 153
  Speedy Miso Noodle Soup, 173
  Starter Guacamole, 73
  Sweet Carrot Salad, 31
  Taco-Spiced Skillet Chickpeas, 139
  Very Berry Pops, 147
Refried beans, 192
Resistant starch, 52, 74
Resveratrol, 90
Riboflavin, 64, 140, 156
Rice, 118–119, 132
Rice milk, 165
Road trips, foods for, 198
Roasted broccoli, 22
Rolled oats, 126
Romaine lettuce, 56
Rutin, 18

S

Salad dressings, 170
Salads
  Caesar, 56
  cucumber, 38
  Sweet Carrot Salad, 31
Salmon, 170–171, 196
Salt, 97
Saturated fat, 61, 84, 144, 178
Sauerkraut, 29
Seedless melons, 113
Selenium, 49, 166
Semisweet chocolate, 178
Sesame seeds, 168
Skin, apple, 68
Smoothies, 21, 75, 77, 86, 143
Snacks/snacking
  benefits of, 101
  edamame, 148
  packaged fruit, 71
  peanuts, 158
  pistachios, 155
  providing filling, 117
  veggie chips and, 41
Soluble fiber, 102, 126, 136, 163
Sorbitol, 107
Soy milk, 145
Spinach, 57, 77, 194
Split lentils, 152
Stearic acid, 178
Steel-cut oats, 126
Strawberries, 194
  Berry and Beet Smoothie, 21
  Melted Berry Sauce, 111
Sugar(s)
  coconut, 85
  in dates, 86
  guidelines on limits for, 71
  honey replaced for white, 185
  in juice, 69
  on labels, 103
  reducing in your child's diet, 87
  in store-bought applesauce, 69
  in yogurt, 146
Sulfur dioxide, 83
Sunflower seed butter, 166
Sunflower seeds, 166–167
Sweet peppers, 58–59
Sweet potatoes, 60–61, 194
Synthetic food dyes, 191

T

Tabbouleh, 120
Tahini, 168–169

Teeth cleaners, 133
Thirst, 117
Tofu, 172–173, 193
Tomatoes, 62–63
Trail mix, 195, 198
"Try it" tips
  beef, 137
  broccoli, 23
  Brussels sprouts, 25
  carrots, 31
  cauliflower, 33
  celery, 35
  cinnamon, 181
  cottage cheese, 141
  cucumbers, 39
  eggplant, 41
  fruit kebabs, 81
  garlic, 183
  grapes, 91
  kiwifruit, 92
  lentils, 154
  peanut butter, 159
  prunes/dried plums, 107
  quinoa, 129
  salmon, 171
  smoothies, 77
  sweet peppers, 59
  tofu, 173
  tomatoes, 63
  turmeric, 191
  walnuts, 161
  whole wheat pasta, 131
Tuna, 174–175, 196
Turmeric, 190–191

U
Umami taste sense, 49
Unsaturated fat, 156

V
Valencia oranges, 98
Vegan diet, 128, 165, 186
Vegetables. See also specific names of
    vegetables
  cut into different shapes and sizes, 31
  recommended daily intake, 17
  resistance to eating, 35
  sneaking into recipes, 65
  tips for keeping fresh, 27
Vegetarian diet, 128, 149, 186

Veggie chips, 31, 197
Vitamin A, 22, 26, 30, 36, 44, 54, 61, 62,
    80, 84, 94, 95, 100, 112, 140
Vitamin B_6, 20, 64, 70, 137, 160
Vitamin B_{12}, 137, 140, 174
Vitamin C, 18, 19, 20, 22, 24, 26, 28, 32,
    34, 36, 44, 45, 48, 49, 52, 56, 58, 62,
    64, 68, 74, 76, 78, 79, 80, 82, 88, 92,
    93, 94, 95, 98, 100, 102, 104, 106, 108,
    110, 112
Vitamin D, 49, 51, 84, 98, 121, 141, 142, 144,
    145, 165
Vitamin E, 70, 130, 156, 166
Vitamin K, 18, 38, 42, 57, 64, 90, 188

W
Walnuts, 160–161
Watermelon, 112–113
"Wheat" bread, 197
White button mushrooms, 137
White chocolate, 178
White rice, 118
Whole grain barley, 116
Whole grain crackers, 198, 199
Whole milk, 144
Whole wheat, 130
Whole wheat pasta, 192
Wild blueberries, 79, 196
Wild-caught salmon, 170–171
Wild rice, 132

Y
Yams, 60
Yogurt, 74, 99, 146–147, 194, 195, 199

Z
Zeaxanthin, 56, 57
"Zebra Pasta," 131
Zinc, 16, 120, 125, 137, 138, 164, 166
Zucchini, 64